your guide to breast cancer

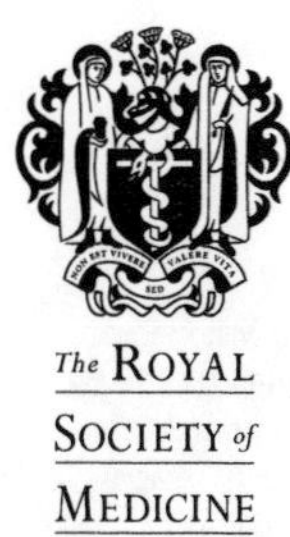

your guide to breast cancer

Jacqueline Lewis
FRCS (Glasg), FRCS (Plast)

Hodder Arnold
A MEMBER OF THE HODDER HEADLINE GROUP

Orders: Please contact Bookpoint Ltd, 130 Milton Park, Abingdon, Oxon OX14 4SB. Telephone: (44) 01235 827720. Fax: (44) 01235 400454. Lines are open from 9.00 to 18.00, Monday to Saturday, with a 24-hour message answering service. You can also order through our website www.hoddereducation.com

British Library Cataloguing in Publication Data
A catalogue record for this title is available from the British Library.

ISBN-10: 0 340 90500 X
ISBN-13: 9 780340 905005

First published	2005
Impression number	10 9 8 7 6 5 4 3 2 1
Year	2008 2007 2006 2005

Typeset by Servis Filmsetting Limited, Longsight, Manchester. Printed in Great Britain for Hodder Arnold, a division of Hodder Headline, 338 Euston Road, London NW1 3BH, by Cox & Wyman Ltd, Reading, Berkshire.

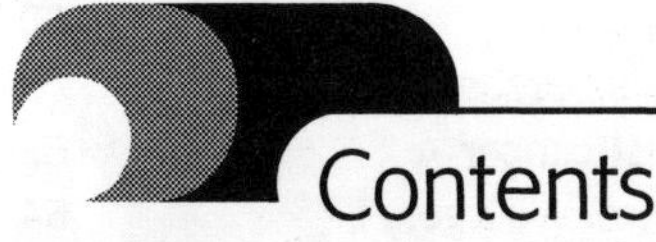

Contents

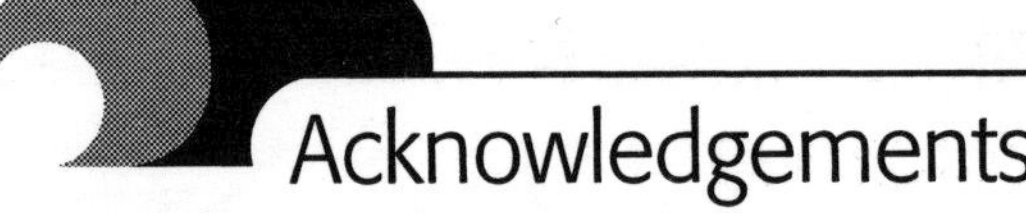

Acknowledgements

The author and publishers would like to thank the following:

Charles Lowdell
Alyson Dyer
Mark Harries
Addie Mitchell
Ann Alexander
Shelagh Wilson
Sami Shousha
Anthony Alwyn
Keshthra Satchithananda
Felicity Muncey
Vanessa Cross
Donald McRobbie
Dudley Sinnett
Charles Coombes
Tony Dhillon
Judith Hughes
Simon Eccles
Nikki Kettley
Maria Fernandez

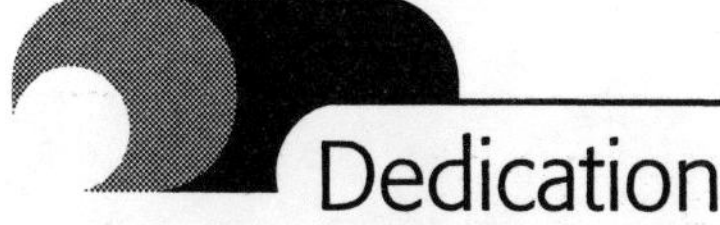

Dedication

For Mummy, Wendy and Philip

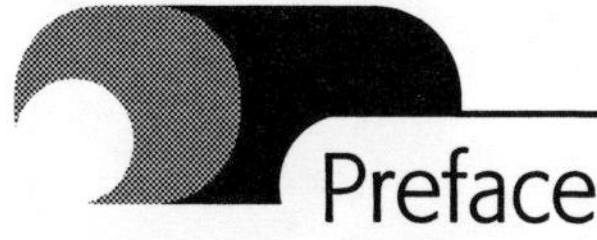

Preface

This new book, published in partnership with the Royal Society of Medicine, provides detailed, useful and up-to-date information on breast cancer. It contains expert yet user-friendly advice, with such useful features as:

Key Terms: demystifying the jargon
Questions and Answers: answering the burning questions
Myths and Facts: debunking the misconceptions
My Experience: how it feels to live with, or care for someone with, this condition.

Bearing the hallmark of excellence and accessibility that characterizes the work of the Royal Society of Medicine, this important guide will enable you and your family to gain some control over the way your breast cancer is managed by being better informed.

Peter Richardson
Director of Publications
Royal Society of Medicine

Introduction

This book is aimed at all those women and men who have, in some way, been touched by breast cancer. It may be you, your wife, mother sister, daughter, another relation or a friend. Nearly all of us know someone who has it, or has had it. Breast cancer is a common disease. It is to be taken seriously. This book is also for those women who are disease free so that they may educate themselves about breast cancer, know what to look out for and seek advice at an early stage. The key to survival is early detection.

I see my mother, close friends and patients live full lives with breast cancer, having gone through the process of diagnosis and treatment. Seeing how they cope, along with my knowledge of the disease and of the available treatments and reconstructive options, reassures me. The routine of examining my breasts on a monthly basis, and being 'breast aware', is now part of my ritual.

Managing breast cancer now is not just about saving a life or saving a breast. It is about achieving the best quality of life, living with the disease and getting the most acceptable cosmetic result with the various available treatment methods. It is also about helping women to make decisions about their sometimes complex choices.

Breast cancer affects many more women than men. Ninety-nine out of every 100 cases of breast cancer occur in women rather than men, and it is for this reason that I have taken the liberty of using the term 'women' when speaking of breast cancer patients. Breast cancer in men is just as important, and men should be aware that they could develop it too. The presentation and treatment of breast cancer in men is much the same as for women and any differences are mentioned in the relevant sections in this book.

This book is dedicated to those women and men with breast cancer who have shown me that it is possible to 'live' with this disease rather than suffer from it, or have to battle with it. It has been an inspiration to me, working with you to get through your diagnosis, treatment and follow-up. My hope is that the information in this book will empower you, the reader, to get involved with breast cancer management, to ask the questions you want the answers to and to tell your doctors, nurses and carers what matters most to you.

CHAPTER 1

Why do people get breast cancer?

Incidence

Cancer is a common disease. One in three people can expect a diagnosis of some form of cancer in their lifetime. In the UK, breast cancer is the most common cancer in women and the most common cause of cancer death in women. About 1 in 9 women can expect to develop breast cancer in their lifetime. There are about 41,000 new female cases of breast cancer diagnosed per year. However there are only about 42 deaths per 100,000 women per year from breast cancer in the general population.

Despite these numbers, women are benefiting from improvements in detecting and treating breast cancer, with death rates falling faster in the UK than anywhere else in the world. While it is such a common disease, there are many women who are alive and live a full life with a diagnosis of breast cancer. It is estimated that there are over 170,000 women alive in the UK

Q What does the 1 in 9 in a lifetime figure mean?

A If a woman lives to the age of 90, there is a 12 per cent chance that she will have a diagnosis of breast cancer in her lifetime. Most women die from causes other than breast cancer, such as coronary heart disease or stroke.

who have been diagnosed with breast cancer in the previous ten years.

The incidence of breast cancer is different around the world with the highest rates occurring in women living in the developed Western world and the lowest numbers in women living in the Far East. Current knowledge suggests that there are many different factors that influence the incidence of breast cancer. They are probably a combination of environmental and inherited factors. The incidence of breast cancer is much lower in Japan than in the UK, USA and Australia despite similar economic success. This suggests that the economy of a country has no influence on the incidence of breast cancer. Yet the incidence of breast cancer can rise when an individual migrates from an area of low risk to high risk.

Causes and risk factors

There are various factors that put women more at risk or reduce the risk of breast cancer. For some of these risk factors there is not much that can be done to change them, for example, getting old and being female. However, women can adopt a healthy lifestyle and reduce known risk factors. Women should also be 'breast aware' and examine their own breasts regularly, every month, so that they will know if there is a change in their breasts. They can also have regular mammograms on the National Health Service (NHS) Breast Screening Programme. 'Breast awareness' is covered in Chapter 2 (see page 45).

The causes of breast cancer can be divided into three main groups:

1 Sporadic
2 Familial
3 Hereditary.

Sporadic

Most (up to eight out of ten) breast cancers occur at random, and these are called sporadic. This is where there is a spontaneous change in a gene in a certain cell, and when that one cell is affected, it can become a cancerous cell. The affected cell will divide and multiply unlike the other cells with normal genes. It is not known what causes the changes in 'sporadic' breast cancer. Most likely, the changes are caused by different factors relating to what the woman is exposed to in the environment or the actions from the chemical messengers (hormones) in the blood.

Hereditary

Breast cancer that is passed on from a parent to a child only accounts for fewer than one in ten of all breast cancers (see page 6 and Chapter 2, page 43).

Familial

The rest of breast cancers, about one in five, are 'familial'. This means they can be attributed to faulty genes which are prominent in certain families. While there are more cases of breast cancer in these certain families than usual, there is no definite pattern of how the faulty gene is passed from parent to child.

The risk factors for breast cancer

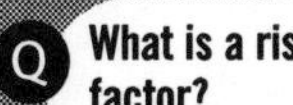

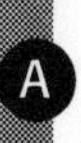

Q What is a risk factor?

A 'Risk factor' in breast cancer refers to a characteristic or exposure that relates to the likelihood of developing breast cancer.

Various risk factors are listed below and divided according to whether they reduce or increase the risk of breast cancer.

Factors that increase the risk of breast cancer:

- Country of birth (developed country)
- Increasing age

- Female sex
- Having had a breast cancer
- Family history of breast cancer
- Abnormal breast tissue on biopsy
- Nodular densities (shadowing) on mammogram
- High dose radiation to chest
- Prolonged oestrogen exposure
- Smoking
- Excessive weight
- Heavy alcohol intake
- Urban place of residence and social class
- Race/ethnicity.

Q What does 'relative risk' mean?

A This is a term used in epidemiological studies (studies of populations) of risk factors. For breast cancer, it is the rate of breast cancer in the 'exposed' population divided by the rate in the 'unexposed' or general population. For example, if a woman has a relative risk of 1.5 times because she drinks more than six units of alcohol per week, it means that her risk of breast cancer is 50 per cent higher than (or 1.5 times) the risk of women who drink less than that amount.

Country of birth (developed country)

Women are at a higher risk of developing breast cancer if they are born in Northern America or Northern Europe; women are at lower risk if they are born in Asia or Africa. Women who move from a low-risk to a high-risk area ultimately take on the risk of the new area. It appears that the earlier in life a woman takes up residence in a 'high-risk' country, the higher her risk of breast cancer compared to that of her country of origin. For example, a Japanese girl moving to North America will have the higher risk of American women rather than the lower risk of Japanese women.

Increasing age

Eighty per cent of women who are diagnosed with breast cancer in the UK are over the age of 50. Half of all breast cancers are found in women between the ages of 50–64 years. One of the reasons is because at this age most women have their first mammogram on the NHS Breast Screening Programme. Breast cancer is uncommon in women under the age of 30.

The table below shows an estimate of the risk of developing breast cancer by age.

Table 1 An estimate of the risk of developing breast cancer by age

Risk up to age 25	1 in 15,000 women
Risk up to age 30	1 in 1,900
Risk up to age 40	1 in 200
Risk up to age 50	1 in 50
Risk up to age 60	1 in 23
Risk up to age 70	1 in 15
Risk up to age 80	1 in 11
Risk up to age 85	1 in 10
Lifetime risk (all ages)	1 in 9

Source: Breast Cancer Factsheet, February 2004, Cancer Research UK.

Female sex

Being female is a definite risk factor for getting breast cancer. Ninety-nine per cent of all breast cancers occur in women. Breast cancer does occur in men too but it is rare (about 1 per cent). In the UK, the incidence of male breast cancer is 1 in 100,000 with about 290 new cases of male breast cancer diagnosed per year (as compared with 41,000 female breast cancers). Risk factors for male breast cancer are carrying an altered or

BRCA1, BRCA2 and TP53 genes
Genes that if altered or faulty put an individual at an increased risk of breast and other types of cancer. They can be passed from one generation to the next.

TP53
A cancer gene also known as tumour protein p53 (Li-Fraumeni syndrome). It is a tumour suppressor gene and acts by regulating the cycle of cell division by preventing cells from dividing and growing in an uncontrolled way.

gynaecomastia
Male breast enlargement.

faulty breast cancer gene (**BRCA1**, **BRCA2**, **TP53**), previous radiotherapy to the chest and, less importantly, **gynaecomastia**, undescended testis, obesity, and an increased exposure to oestrogen.

Having had a breast cancer

Women with a treated cancer in one breast have a five-fold increased risk of a cancer arising in their other breast when compared with the general population. This means that about 1 in every 100 women with breast cancer develop cancer in the opposite breast every year. Women should therefore check their breasts every month and report any new changes in their breasts. All cancer centres have a follow-up protocol for women who have been treated for breast cancer (see Chapter 4, page 123)

Family history of breast cancer

We know that certain breast cancer genes that are passed down from generation to generation in certain families can cause breast cancer. When a breast cancer gene is inherited and an individual develops breast cancer, the cancer is considered to be 'hereditary'. This is not a common cause of breast cancer. Families in which there are many members who have breast cancer are more likely to carry an altered or faulty breast cancer gene but only about 3 per cent of families with a history of breast cancer carry a gene. A parent does not always pass a faulty gene to their child. The chance of passing it on is 1 in 2 (50 per cent chance).

BRCA1 and BRCA2 genes

BRCA1 and BRCA2 are genes known to be associated with breast cancer. Women who inherit a faulty BRCA1 or BRCA2 gene have an increased lifetime risk of breast, ovarian and possibly colon (large bowel) cancer. Men are also at a higher risk of breast cancer (more so with BRCA2) and possibly prostate cancer. Testing for these genes is possible but not entirely accurate, and there are many other, yet to be discovered, genes that probably cause breast cancer.

Carrying a faulty breast cancer gene does not necessarily mean that a woman will get breast cancer. A mutation of the gene in the breast is what causes the breast cancer to develop. This is why some women who carry the predisposing gene live their entire life without developing breast cancer. It is also the reason why the identical twin of a woman (who has identical genes to her twin) with breast cancer may never develop it. The lifetime risks are estimated at 60–90 per cent. The differences in the estimated rates are large because different populations and different gene mutations were studied to result in this estimation. Breast cancers tend to occur at a younger age in women who carry faulty BRCA1 or BRCA2 genes.

In the general population, it is estimated that 1 in 800 women carry the faulty BRCA1 gene. There is a higher incidence of genetic mutations in both BRCA1 and BRCA2 genes in women of Ashkenazi Jewish descent, and so these women are at a higher risk of breast and ovarian cancer.

Abnormal breast tissue on biopsy

Abnormal breast tissue is usually found when a woman has a **core biopsy** for a breast abnormality which has been found on screening. The risks outlined below for each condition do not remain constant throughout a woman's lifetime. For example, the relative risk of breast cancer in women with atypical hyperplasia (ductal or lobular) goes down the longer they remain free of breast cancer.

core (needle) biopsy
A type of thick needle biopsy where a small core of tissue is removed from an area in the breast without surgery.

atypical ductal hyperplasia
Cells lining a breast duct that are slightly abnormal and increased in number.

atypical lobular hyperplasia
Abnormal cells within a breast lobule that are increased in number but fill less than half of the acini.

lobular carcinoma in situ (LCIS)
Abnormal cells within a breast lobule (part of the breast capable of producing milk) that fill, distend and distort more than half the acini of a breast lobule. This serves as a marker for future breast cancer risk.

radial scar
A radial scar is a benign (non-cancerous) area of fibrous tissue surrounded by breast glands, some of which may look abnormal under the microscope. On a mammogram a radial scar has the appearance of having long spicules (strands) radiating from a central area. A lump is not usually palpable in the breast.

Atypical ductal hyperplasia

A woman who has **atypical ductal hyperplasia** (ADH), without a family history of breast cancer, has a four-fold increased risk of breast cancer. This risk is doubled if she has a family history of breast cancer in a first-degree relative (mother, sister, daughter). The risk of breast cancer is bilateral (equally likely to occur in either breast).

Atypical lobular hyperplasia

Women with **atypical lobular hyperplasia** (ALH) have an increased risk of breast cancer similar to that of having ADH (see above).

Lobular carcinoma in situ

Lobular carcinoma in situ (LCIS) is a marker for breast cancer; it identifies women at an increased risk for subsequently developing invasive cancer. However, despite the term 'carcinoma' in its name, it is not a cancer in the true sense of the word. The risk of developing a cancer in either breast is about 1 per cent per year. Both breasts are at equal risk of developing a cancer. The risk is greater where there is a positive family history of breast cancer.

Radial scar

The risk of breast cancer in women who have a **radial scar** is double that of the normal population.

myth
I am afraid that I am at an increased risk of breast cancer because I have lumpy breasts and I have been told that I have benign fibrocystic changes in my breasts.

fact
Benign fibrocystic change does not increase the risk of breast cancer.

Nodular densities (shadowing) on mammogram

Studies have shown that women with a high proportion of dense tissue on their mammogram have a two to four times increased risk of breast cancer. This may be because ADH and ALH are more common in dense breasts.

High dose radiation to the chest

High dose radiation to the chest (radiotherapy) is associated with an increased risk of breast cancer especially if the exposure was at a young age (between puberty and age 30). Patients treated for **Hodgkin's disease** (cancer of the lymph nodes) in this manner have a three to eight times increased risk of breast cancer depending on the dose of radiation to the chest and ovaries, and whether or not chemotherapy was given at that time. The risk is higher with increased doses of radiotherapy to the chest wall. The risks are reduced with modern radiotherapy techniques and lower doses of radiotherapy that reduce the amount of breast tissue exposed. There are guidelines that detail the recommended investigations – mammogram or breast ultrasound or magnetic resonance imaging (MRI) scan – for women having had radiotherapy for Hodgkin's disease according to their age, appearance of their breasts on mammography and whether or not they can tolerate MRI scanning. Women should ask their oncologist or general practitioner for a referral to a breast unit to assess their risk and for any necessary investigations.

> **Hodgkin's disease**
> A type of cancer involving the lymph nodes.

Prolonged oestrogen exposure

Women have natural oestrogens circulating around their body, and throughout a woman's lifetime there are cyclical changes of the levels of oestrogens. At puberty and when menstruation starts (**menarche**), there is a surge in the

> **menarche**
> Age at which menstruation or a woman's periods starts.

menopause
'Change of life', the time in a woman's life when her periods stop and her ovaries stop producing oestrogen.

amount of circulating oestrogens. These levels rise and fall on a monthly basis until the **menopause**. After the menopause, the ovaries stop producing oestrogen but there is still some oestrogen produced by other tissues to a smaller extent. When a woman becomes pregnant, there is a massive surge of hormones, including oestrogen, in order to maintain the pregnancy.

A woman cannot really control the age at which her periods will naturally start or stop. She can, however, plan to a certain extent at what age she would like to start a family, whether or not to breastfeed, and she can choose the amount of exposure to exogenous oestrogens like taking HRT or the oral contraceptive pill.

endogenous oestrogen
Oestrogen that is produced within the woman's own body.

Endogenous oestrogen

Age at menarche and menopause

Studies have shown that women who start their periods at or before the age of 11 have a higher risk of developing breast cancer compared to women who started their periods at age 14 or older. Also, women who have their menopause at a later age (after 50 years of age) have a higher risk of breast cancer than those women who have an early menopause.

Most of the evidence for the role of oestrogens in breast cancer is from studies on women who have had an artificially induced menopause caused by the removal of one or both ovaries. After **ovarian ablation**, the risk of breast cancer can be significantly reduced, with the greatest risk reduction seen in young, thin women who have not had children.

ovarian ablation
Suppression of oestrogen production by the ovaries or surgical removal of the ovaries.

A number of studies suggest that oestrogen levels are higher in women who develop breast cancer than in those who do not. It has been shown that oestrogen levels can be decreased with maintenance of ideal body weight and a low-fat diet in post-menopausal women and moderate exercise in adolescent girls. The evidence does not suggest that all women need to have their oestrogen levels checked. However, it would seem sensible for all women to eat a well-balanced diet and to exercise regularly in order to live a healthy life and at the same time reduce their risk of developing breast cancer.

First full-term pregnancy after 30 years and never having a full-term pregnancy

Women who start their family before the age of 20 are half as likely to develop breast cancer, compared to women who have not had any children or who have their first child at 35 years or older. A woman who has never had children has approximately the same risk as a woman who has her first baby around the age of 30. There is a transient increase in risk of breast cancer in the first three to four years after delivery of a baby. Subsequently though, women who have had children have a lower lifetime risk of breast cancer than women who have not had children.

Exogenous oestrogen

HRT

There is good evidence to show that there is a definite increased risk of breast cancer for women who take any type of **Hormone Replacement Therapy (HRT)**. This risk increases within one to two years of starting HRT and is related to the length of time that HRT is used. The longer a woman uses HRT, the higher the risk of breast cancer.

HRT should not be taken for any other reasons apart from improving post-menopausal symptoms such as vaginal dryness or soreness, headaches and hot flushes. When used, HRT should be used at the minimum effective dose for the shortest duration. Tibolone (Livial®) is a

Exogenous oestrogen
Oestrogen from an external source like the contraceptive pill or HRT.

Hormone Replacement Therapy (HRT)
Drugs containing oestrogen with or without progesterone that are used to treat the symptoms of menopause.

synthetic steroid drug that is used to relieve menopausal symptoms. It also increases the risk of breast cancer. While HRT does reduce post-menopausal osteoporosis (thinning/ softening of bones), other medications are recommended instead of HRT.

myth
HRT has a protective effect on the heart.

fact
HRT does not reduce the incidence of coronary heart disease and should not be used for this purpose.

Q What is the risk of breast cancer for women taking HRT?

Approximately 32 in every 1000 women (aged between 50–65) who will get breast cancer if they do not take HRT. An extra 19 per 1000 women will get breast cancer after having used HRT for ten years if they used the combined oestrogen and progesterone HRT. For women using oestrogen only HRT, the risk is less but still higher than women who do not use HRT. The excess risk disappears within about five years of stopping HRT.

Oral contraceptives

Oral contraceptives ('the pill') are contraindicated (not advised) in women with breast cancer. Older preparations of the oral contraceptive pill contained larger doses of oestrogen. Women on older preparations of oral contraceptives had a small increased risk of breast cancer compared to women who had never used them. The risk of breast cancer reduced after stopping 'the pill' and was the same as non-users after ten years. Studies looking at whether or not modern preparations that contain less oestrogen cause an increased risk of breast cancer are underway.

Fertility treatment

Multiple stimulated cycles for fertility treatment cause marked elevations in the levels of circulating oestrogens. There is no evidence at present to show whether there is an increased risk of breast cancer with this treatment. Studies are being carried out to try to answer this question.

Smoking

There is some evidence to show that there is an increased risk of breast cancer in pre-menopausal women who smoke. The risk of breast cancer is related to the number of cigarettes smoked and the length of time that women have smoked. The increased risk seems to go down when women stop smoking. Further studies are being carried out to validate these findings.

Excessive weight

Obesity is associated with an increased risk of breast cancer in post-menopausal women if they have not used HRT. In women who are overweight when they are first diagnosed with breast cancer, the risk of the breast cancer recurring increases by as much as five times.

Heavy alcohol intake

There is about a 50 per cent increased risk of breast cancer in women who drink more than five to six units of alcohol per week. The type of alcoholic drink does not seem to influence the risk. A unit of alcohol (8 gm or 10 ml of alcohol) is equivalent to one small glass of wine, a half pint of ordinary beer, lager or cider, one measure of fortified wine (port or whisky) or a single measure of spirits. In practical terms, it has been estimated that if 1000 women over the age of 30 maintained a moderate regular intake of alcohol for two years, there would be one extra case of breast cancer. The quality of life issue has to be balanced considering that the risk from alcohol in moderation is small. Furthermore, there is a potential benefit from drinking alcohol in moderation for the reduction of heart disease.

Urban place of residence and social class

The risk of breast cancer is greater (up to two times) in women from higher socio-economic classes and in women who live in an urban area as opposed to a rural area.

my experience

At the age of 41 years, two years ago, I discovered that I was one of the 'one in nine' women who get breast cancer. The statistics hide thousands of very different personal stories. 'Why me?' I asked. I knew of no women in my family who had had cancer before me and I seemed to belong to none of the risk groups which we so regularly hear about nowadays.
The diagnosis came soon after I stopped breastfeeding my child. The most joyous and potentially the most tragic of aspects of being a woman came so close together that they forced me to think about women's lives – including my own – in a very different light.

Race/ethnicity

Caucasians and Blacks have a higher risk (up to two times) of breast cancer than Asians. This may be related to diet and because Asian women tend to start their menstruation at a later age.

Factors that reduce the risk of breast cancer:

- Losing excess weight
- Reducing alcohol intake
- Minimizing or eliminating oestrogen
- Not smoking
- Eating a healthy diet
- Breastfeeding
- Regular exercise
- Rural place of residence.

The protective benefits from losing excess weight, reducing alcohol intake, minimizing exposure to excess oestrogens and not smoking are not only confined to breast cancer but to a whole host of other diseases. The risks from each have been detailed above.

Eating a healthy diet

Most studies have looked at women with a diagnosis of breast cancer and the risk of relapse. About half of all studies that looked at the risk of breast cancer and diet show that diets high in fruit and vegetables lowered the risk of dying from breast cancer. There is no clear evidence to show a link between the amount and type of dietary fat or fibre and breast cancer recurrence. There is some evidence to suggest that a diet high in fish oils may be protective. A diet rich in vitamins A and C, folate and beta-carotene may reverse the increased risk associated with alcohol use. There is no evidence to show that dietary red meat has any effect on the risk of breast cancer. Phytoestrogens are naturally occurring plant compounds that are converted to oestrogen in the gut. They are found in soybean products and other health food supplements. There is a lower incidence of breast cancer in women who live in the East where soybean products are widely used. Large trials are needed to tell us whether phytoestrogens have a protective effect against breast cancer.

Breastfeeding

Breastfeeding is associated with a slight reduction in the risk of breast cancer, and the most benefit is found in pre-menopausal women at a young age. This protective effect seems to be best for women who have had long periods of breastfeeding during their lifetime. There does not seem to be a benefit for post-menopausal women who have breastfed their children. A woman who has been breastfed herself may also be protected against breast cancer, however, the evidence for this is not strong.

Regular exercise

There is evidence to show that regular exercise reduces the risk of breast cancer. The benefit is greatest in women under the age of 45.

The amount of exercise necessary in order to benefit has yet to be worked out. It appears that doing three to four hours of physical activity per week over many years is beneficial.

Preventative measures for women at high risk of developing breast cancer

The main measures available for preventing breast cancer in women at high risk are the use of medications (drugs) that reduce the effects of circulating oestrogens in the body, and preventative surgery. The preventative surgical options available are the surgical removal of the breast tissue (risk-reducing mastectomy), or the surgical removal of the ovaries (risk-reducing oophorectomy).

Medications

Selective Oestrogen Receptor Modulators

Selective Oestrogen Receptor Modulators (SERMs) are drugs that reduce the effect of circulating oestrogens in the body. One such drug is tamoxifen. There is evidence to show that tamoxifen reduces the risk of developing breast cancer in women who are at a high risk. The estimated reduction in risk is 50 per cent. Because tamoxifen does have side effects (see Chapter 4, page 106), each individual woman should carefully weigh up the risks versus the potential benefits of using tamoxifen.

Preventative surgery

Risk-reducing mastectomy

Risk-reducing mastectomy involves the surgical removal of the breast(s) in order to prevent or reduce the occurrence of breast cancer. For women who carry a faulty breast cancer gene, for example BRCA1 or BRCA2, **bilateral prophylactic mastectomy** (removing both breasts) reduces the risk of breast cancer by as much as 90 per cent. However, it cannot completely eliminate the risk. Mastectomy is an irreversible procedure and has physical and psychological effects, and consequently a decision to have this surgery is not to be taken lightly. Mastectomy results in loss (or reduced) of sensation of the chest wall. Immediate breast reconstruction is usually offered at the same time. Women should know and understand their individual risk and be counselled before considering this option.

bilateral prophylactic mastectomy
Surgical removal of both breasts in order to reduce the risk of a breast cancer.

myth
The risk of breast cancer is completely eliminated with bilateral prophylactic mastectomy.

fact
Not all of the breast tissue can be removed by mastectomy. For women at high risk, the risk can be reduced by up to 90 per cent but this surgery cannot completely eliminate the risk.

Risk-reducing oophorectomy

There is about a 50 per cent reduction in the risk of developing breast cancer in BRCA1 mutation carriers if a risk-reducing oophorectomy (surgical removal of ovaries) procedure is carried out before the natural menopause. However, there is an increased risk of osteoporosis, heart disease and reduced quality of life because of the loss of oestrogen that this procedure causes in the long term.

myth
Using antiperspirants causes breast cancer.

fact
A message on the internet some time ago worried many women about the use of antiperspirants. The use of antiperspirants is common. Breast cancer is common. There is more breast tissue in the upper outer half of the breasts, and breast cancers commonly occur in that area. The lymphatic drainage from breast gland tissue mostly goes in the direction of the lymph nodes in the armpit (it also goes to the nodes beside the breastbone). Lymphatic drainage from the breast goes away from the breast, not towards it. There is no evidence to show that substances that block sweat release from the armpit move into the breast. No convincing evidence exists to show that there is a link between the use of antiperspirants and breast cancer.

Factors that do not cause an increased risk of breast cancer

Stress

While stress causes hormonal levels to rise and fall, there is no evidence to date to show that it is related to breast cancer.

Abortion

There is good evidence to show that abortions (spontaneous or induced) are not associated with an increased risk of breast cancer.

Factors currently under study

Environmental contaminants

It is not known whether environmental contaminants, like pesticides, increase breast cancer risk.

Maternal exposure to oestrogen

There is a question about whether maternal exposure to high doses of oestrogen (for example, the drug diethyl stilboestrol that was used for pregnant women in order to prevent miscarriage) is associated with an increase in breast cancer risk in the daughters. There is no evidence for this at present.

Dairy products

Studies of populations who have a low intake of dairy products show a low incidence of breast cancer. There are conflicting results about whether milk increases or reduces the risk of breast cancer. Dairy products contain many different substances that may promote breast cancer risk or reduce it. Conjugated linoleic acid or (CLA), a substance found in milk, has been suggested to have an effect on reducing the risk. On the other hand, milk increases levels of a growth hormone, IGF-1, in the body, and increased IGF-1 levels have been linked with breast cancer.

Q A lot of women I know have eliminated dairy products from their diet because they feel it will prevent breast cancer. Should I do that too?

A We still do not have enough information about dairy products and breast cancer. Anyone who wishes to eliminate a particular food group from their diet should ensure that they have a substitute that will provide a balanced diet that includes all the minerals, vitamins, essential fatty acids and other essential nutrients from another source. If you exclude dairy food from your diet you need to ensure that you get your calcium and Vitamin D from a different source such as oily fish, margarine, spinach, baked beans and some cereals.

Birth weight

There is a suggestion that birth weight is related to breast cancer risk. Studies have shown that babies who are born weighing more than 3000 g grow up to have an increased risk of breast cancer. It may be related to circulating levels of oestrogen and growth hormones in the mother during pregnancy. More work is needed to verify these findings.

CHAPTER

2 What is breast cancer?

Defining cancer

The word 'cancer' is derived from the Latin word meaning 'crab', and is used to describe a malignant tumour (cancerous growth). A cancer starts when a cell begins to divide and grow in an uncontrolled and abnormal way. The cause of this is not known. Over time, these abnormal cells cluster together to form a tumour.

Breast cancers can be invasive (infiltrating) or non-invasive (in situ):

- Invasive cancers can grow and invade into surrounding tissue and the malignant cells can break away from the original tumour to spread to other parts of the body. These cells can grow to form new tumour deposits that are called metastases or secondary tumours (secondaries).
- Non-invasive breast cancers are confined to the ducts (ductal carcinoma in situ – DCIS) of the breast. When there is abnormal

growth of the cells in the breast lobules and there is no invasion, the condition is called lobular caranoma in situ (LCIS) but it is not considered a true breast cancer. It is treated as a risk factor for breast cancer and the opposite breast is as much at risk as the breast containing LCIS.

Primary cancer

A primary breast cancer is a malignant tumour that arises in the breast. It is derived from cells that make up the breast glandular tissue.

Secondary cancer

When an invasive breast cancer spreads beyond the breast to form tumours in other organs, these tumours are called secondary breast cancers or metastases. The common areas that breast cancer metastases are found are the lung, liver, bone and, less often, the brain. When this happens, the cancer is said to be at an advanced stage. Breast cancer is also said to be at an advanced stage if the tumour is very large (greater than 5 cm) or if it has ulcerated through the skin or if it has invaded the muscles of the chest wall. It is the metastases from a breast cancer that affects survival from the disease.

Histological types

There are many different forms of breast cancer, and they are classified according to their growth pattern and how the cells appear under the microscope. They can be invasive (infiltrating) or non-invasive (in-situ). The term invasive 'ductal' carcinoma is given to most breast cancers that have not got any special features and the rest are of a 'special' type with characteristic patterns of appearance and behaviour. In general, 'special' types are associated with less potential for spread and are associated with a better **prognosis** as compared with invasive ductal carcinomas. The 'special' type cancers make up about one third of all invasive cancers in the breast, the remainder being invasive ductal carcinoma. The next most common invasive type is invasive lobular carcinoma.

prognosis
Forecast of the expected or probable outcome of a disease.

Classification of invasive breast cancers

Special types:

- Tubular/Cribriform
- Mucinous or mucoid
- Lobular
- Medullary
- Papillary.

No special type:

- Commonly known as NST or NOS or invasive ductal carcinoma.

The normal breast

In order to understand breast cancer, it helps to know about the structure and function of the breast (see Colour Plate 1). The breast is made up of fat, glandular tissue and fibrous connective tissue (that hold it all together). The breast is a gland that functions to produce milk for a baby. The glandular tissue is made up of 15–20 ductal-lobular units lined by cells. Each lobule is made up of multiple **acini**. When a woman breastfeeds, milk is produced in the lobules and transferred along the ducts that open on the nipple-areola.

acini
Tiny grape-shaped secretory portions of a gland.

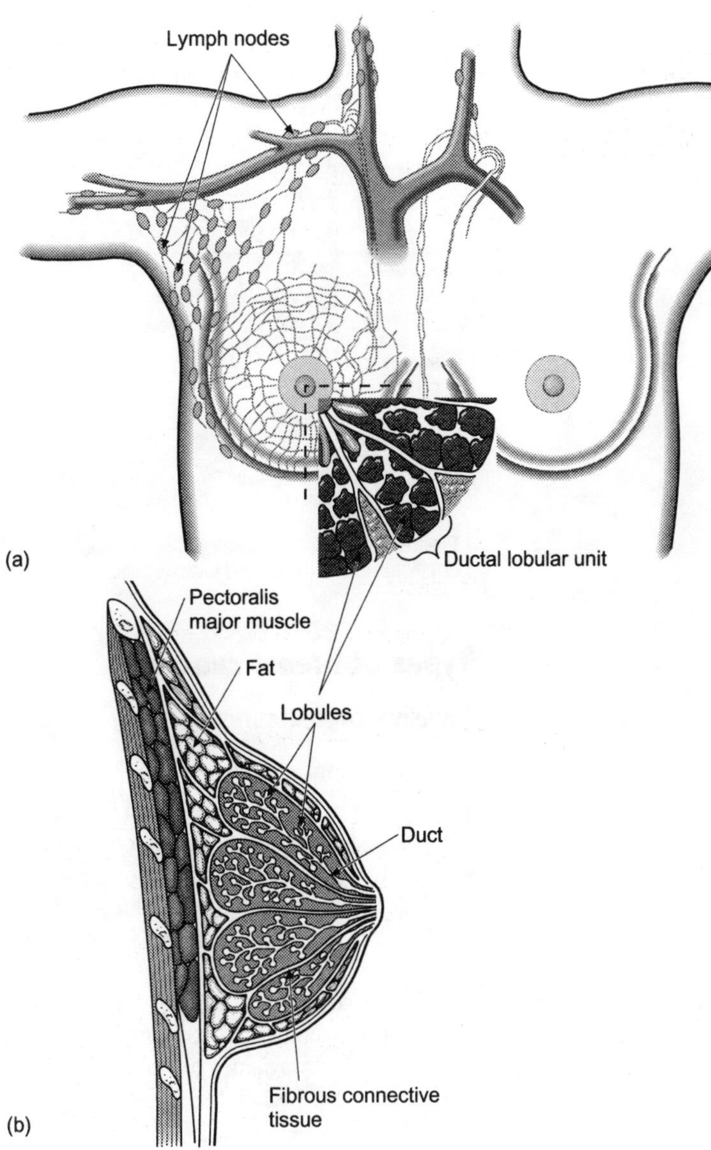

Figure 1 Anatomy of the normal breast.

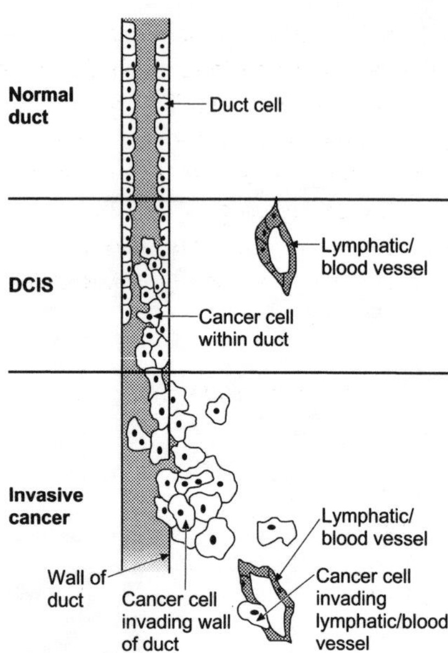

Figure 2 Microscopic anatomy of normal duct, ductal carcinoma in situ (DCIS) and invasive cancer.

Types of breast cancer

Invasive breast cancer

Invasive ductal carcinoma

This is the term given to most breast cancers that are grouped together as 'breast cancer of no special type' NST (or NOS, not otherwise specified). These are called 'ductal' simply because they do not have a lobular pattern and do not show any special type of histologic pattern. This is the commonest type of breast cancer. These cancers commonly occur as a lump, or are seen on a mammogram if too small to feel, or if situated deep within the breast. Prognostic information can be gained by the grade of the tumour. Invasive ductal carcinomas are graded from 1 to 3. Grade 1 tumours are associated with the best outcome and grade 3 with the least favourable outcome. The grading of a tumour depends on how the cells are arranged within the tumour, what they look like and how quickly they are dividing. Most (85 per cent) breast cancers in men are invasive ductal carcinomas whereas in women they account for up to 75 per cent.

Special types of invasive carcinoma

The types of breast cancer in this group include:

- Tubular/Cribriform
- Lobular
- Mucinous or mucoid
- Medullary
- Papillary.

Tubular carcinoma

This is an uncommon form of breast cancer. It rarely metastasises (spreads outside the breast) and the prognosis is excellent. It is most common in older women. The survival rate of patients with tubular carcinoma is similar to that of the general population and systemic adjuvant therapy (therapy such as chemotherapy or hormonal therapy given in addition to primary therapy, usually surgery) is rarely necessary.

Cribriform carcinoma

This is closely related in appearance and behaviour to tubular carcinoma and is associated with a good prognosis.

Lobular carcinoma

This type of cancer is the second most common after invasive ductal carcinoma and arises from cells in the breast lobules. It can cause a thickening rather than a lump in the breast, and is sometimes difficult to feel in the breast or to pick up on a mammogram. Invasive lobular carcinoma is often multifocal (more than one tumour).

Mucinous or mucoid carcinoma

Mucinous (colloid) carcinoma is an uncommon form of invasive breast cancer. It usually affects older women and carries a good prognosis. These tumours characteristically contain mucus (a watery substance).

Medullary carcinoma

Medullary carcinoma has a distinctive smooth border and is seen as a clearly defined mass on a mammogram. It is a common type of hereditary breast cancer in women who carry the altered BRCA1 gene. The prognosis is good for patients who do not have involved lymph nodes.

Papillary carcinoma

Papillary carcinoma is an uncommon form of breast cancer and has a number of different appearances under the microscope. The prognosis is variable.

Unusual types of breast cancer

Inflammatory breast carcinoma

When a breast cancer involves the lymphatic spaces in the dermis (thick middle layer of the skin), there is a characteristic appearance of the breast. The breast appears warm, red and swollen and this is called inflammatory carcinoma. This is an uncommon form of advanced cancer. A lump is not usually felt. The chances of survival to five years is significantly low with an inflammatory breast cancer although **multimodality treatment** with chemotherapy, surgery and radiotherapy may improve survival.

multimodality treatment
The use of different forms of treatment. For breast cancer, surgery, drug therapy and radiotherapy are used.

The unknown primary

One of the commonest ways that the unknown primary breast cancer is diagnosed is by the finding of an enlarged lymph node in the axilla (armpit) that contains cancer cells. If the cancer cells look as if they come from an **adenocarcinoma**, then the likelihood of having a breast cancer is high. In this situation it is common not to feel a lump and sometimes the breast cancer is not easily seen on a mammogram or an ultrasound scan of the breast. The next most useful investigation of the breast would be an MRI scan or PET scan (see pages 51 and 58). Sometimes lymph nodes in the armpit can be involved with lymphoma (cancer of the lymph glands) or skin cancer but they can usually be distinguished on the biopsy appearance of the lymph node.

adenocarcinoma
Cancer that arises in gland-forming tissue. Breast cancer is a type of adenocarcinoma.

Phylloides tumour

Phylloides tumour (cystosarcoma phylloides) is a soft tissue tumour with a very small but definite potential to recur locally and/or metastasise. Histopathology reports will comment on the number of mitoses per high power field (how active the tumour cells look under the microscope) and the appearance of the tumour under the microscope, giving an indication of its malignant potential. The tumours can be classified into benign, borderline (low-grade malignant potential) or malignant. Removing a rim of normal tissue around the tumour will reduce the chance of it recurring. Mastectomy is not usually required unless the tumour is very large in relation to the size of the breast, or when there is a significant risk of the tumour recurring (when part of it is left behind), or if the tumour is classified as malignant. Phylloides tumours that are destined to recur will normally do so within two years of the original diagnosis. Local recurrence does not necessarily mean that it will spread. Many breast recurrences can be successfully re-excised, and most women with local recurrences do not develop metastatic disease.

Non-invasive breast cancer

Non-invasive breast cancers are also known as 'in-situ' cancers where the cells have not invaded through the wall of the breast duct. The main type in this group is ductal carcinoma in situ (DCIS). Paget's disease is usually associated with DCIS. Another 'in-situ' condition is lobular carcinoma in situ that is not considered to be a cancer in the true sense of the word.

Ductal carcinoma in situ

This is an early stage breast cancer. It has not spread beyond the breast ducts, or outside the breast to the lymph nodes or to any other parts of the body (see Colour Plate 2). These cancers are often found on mammography at an early stage. There are several types of DCIS, classified according to their behaviour and their appearance under the microscope (see Colour Plate 3). Some may develop into invasive cancer if they are not removed, although some types may not. As DCIS is a non-invasive cancer, the prognosis is very good and it is highly curable with appropriate treatment.

Microinvasion associated with DCIS is uncommon (less than 1 in 50 cases of DCIS). This is where a very small area is seen under the microscope where the cells have invaded beyond the wall of the duct. Prognosis is very good and has a similar outcome to non-invasive breast cancers.

Lobular carcinoma in situ

This is a non-invasive growth that is confined to the breast lobules. It is not considered to be a cancer in itself but it signifies an increased risk of breast cancer. Women with LCIS have about a 1 per cent risk per year of developing an invasive breast cancer in either breast. Therefore, at 20 years there is a 1 in 5 risk of developing an invasive breast cancer.

Paget's disease

This is a rare form of breast cancer that appears as a moist rash on the nipple and may spread out onto the areola (pigmented skin around the nipple). It is more common in older women. Most cases of Paget's disease of the nipple are associated with DCIS, although some may have an invasive ductal carcinoma deeper within the breast. Prognosis depends on the associated cancer within the breast.

Staging

Tumour stage is the most important predictor of survival from breast cancer. The stage of the breast cancer allows doctors to make the best recommendations for treatment. It also allows for a more accurate comparison of different methods of treatment and their outcomes.

TNM staging system

A standard method for staging that is used throughout the world is called the TNM staging system. 'TNM' stands for 'tumour, nodes and metastases' and the classification is as follows:

- Tumour (T) – largest diameter of the primary tumour.
- Node (N) – lymph node metastasis (whether it has spread to the lymph glands). The node can be either mobile or fixed. When a node is fixed, it is likely that a large proportion of the node is replaced by tumour.
- Metastasis (M) – distant metastasis (whether it has spread anywhere else in the body).

As non-invasive (in situ) cancers do not by definition spread outside the breast, they are classified as Stage 0. Invasive cancers are staged from Stage I–IV.

axillary nodes
Lymph glands in the armpit.

Stage 0 (Early stage)
Non-invasive cancers in the ducts or lobules, or Paget's disease of the nipple.

Stage I (Early stage)

- Tumour is not larger than 2 cm
- Lymph nodes in the axilla do not contain tumour
- No evidence of metastases.

Stage II (Early stage)

- Tumour is not larger than 2 cm but the **axillary nodes** contain tumour
- Tumour is between 2–5 cm, axillary nodes may or may not contain tumour
- Tumour is larger than 5 cm, axillary nodes do not contain tumour
- No evidence of metastases.

Stage III (Advanced stage)

- Tumour is not larger than 5 cm, axillary nodes contain tumour
- Tumour is larger than 5 cm, axillary nodes contain tumour

- Tumour of any size with extension to chest wall and/or skin, any nodal status
- Tumour of any size (with or without extension), **internal mammary nodes** contain tumour
- No evidence of metastases.

Stage IV (Advanced stage)

- Tumour of any size, any node status
- Presence of metastases.

internal mammary nodes
Lymph glands behind the edge of the sternum (breastbone).

Prognosis

The prognosis (outcome) for a woman with a diagnosis of breast cancer is difficult to predict because each woman is different. However, the survival figures for women with different stages of breast cancer are known, and these figures are often quoted as the number of women who survive over a period of five or ten years after their diagnosis (see Figure 3). As it takes time to gather statistics and put them together, the rates that are available to us now will relate to people diagnosed and treated some years ago. The outlook for breast cancer continues to improve, and so figures for women treated more recently may be better.

Survival figures are often quoted as a percentage. For example, women with small cancers measuring less than 2 cm across, with no lymph node involvement and either grade 1 or 2 tumours have an 85–9 per cent survival rate at ten years. This means that 85 to 89 out of every 100 women will live for at least ten years after the diagnosis. A woman will not know if she is likely to be one of the 85 to 89 women who will live or one of the 11 to 15 women who will die from breast cancer in that time. It is worth

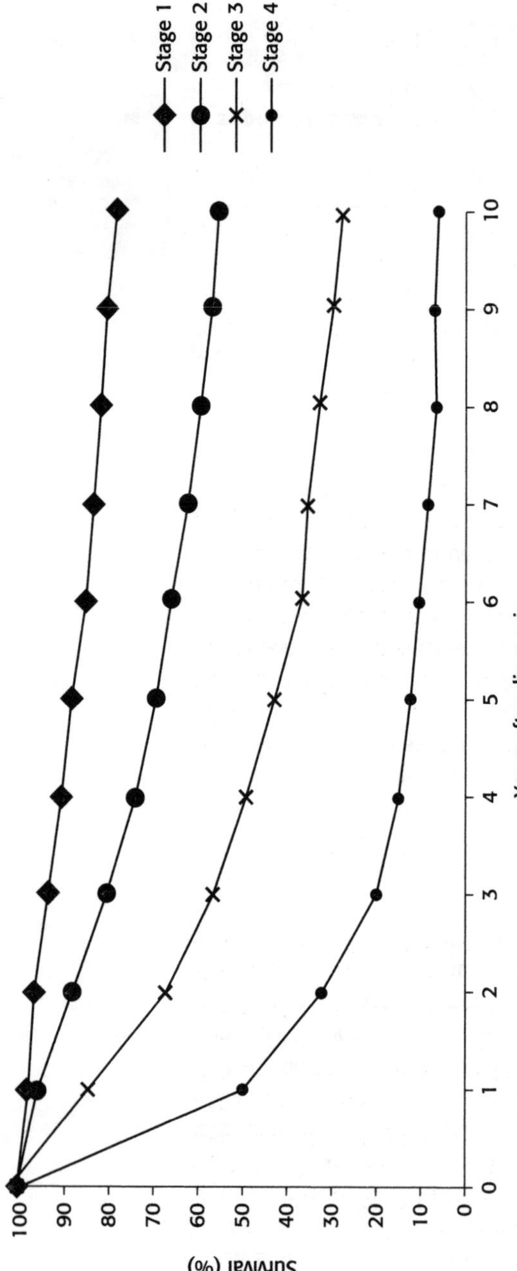

Figure 3 Survival curve according to stage of breast cancer.
Source: Breast Cancer Factsheet, February 2004, Cancer Research UK.

bearing in mind that some of these women will die of a cause unrelated to breast cancer during that period.

The five- or ten-year survival figures do not mean that women will only survive for five or ten years. It is just a point in time after the diagnosis that researchers look at. Studies that quote ten-year survival figures show that more women will have died at ten years as compared with five years, not only from breast cancer but also from other causes. It is therefore important not to attach too much importance to figures. It is also worthwhile remembering that some women may be alive after many years with a recurrence of their breast cancer, and that they continue to live with it.

Disease-free survival figures show the number of women who survive without any evidence of a recurrence of their breast cancer over a period of time. Most breast cancers recur in the first two years after treatment. The likelihood of a cancer recurring after that is much less, and follow-up programmes are designed to take this fact into consideration (see Chapter 4, page 123).

Nottingham Prognostic Index

The Nottingham Prognostic Index is a system used by breast cancer specialists for predicting survival rates and for helping to decide on further treatment. This system was devised by looking at various factors relating to the nature of the tumour and stage of the disease. Three categories for prognosis were identified: good, moderate and poor. It was found that the three most important factors that predict survival after treatment for primary operable breast cancer were the size of the tumour, grade of the invasive

Q I have breast cancer. Will I live?

A Breast cancer is a serious disease. Doctors cannot accurately predict your outcome. All they can do is tell you what has happened in the past to women who have had a similar sort of tumour at a similar stage as yours. There are several indicators of what your outcome may be. These include your general health, age, type and size of breast cancer, and how far the disease has progressed. For example, for early stage breast cancer where no lymph glands are involved with the tumour, the ten-year survival rate is 95 per cent. This means that 95 out of 100 women will survive ten years after their diagnosis, whether their cancers recur or not. It is reasonable to wonder if you will be one of the 95 women who will live the ten years, or one of the five women who will die. No one can tell. Coming to terms with uncertainty is not easy. A lot of women say that they cope by 'living today' (see page 155 for a list of support organizations).

cancer and number of involved lymph nodes. The Nottingham City Hospital breast group has reported long-term survival figures for over 1600 women treated for primary operable breast cancer. The survival rate at 15 years for women in the good prognosis group was 80 per cent, in the moderate prognosis group 42 per cent and in the poor prognosis group 13 per cent.

The NPI formula is calculated as follows:

$$\text{NPI} = (0.2 \times \text{tumour diameter in centimetres}) + \text{lymph node stage} + \text{tumour grade}$$

Scoring system

Lymph node stage

No nodes involved	1
Up to 3 nodes involved	2
More than 3 nodes involved	3

Tumour grade

Grade 1 (less aggressive appearance)	1
Grade 2 (intermediate appearance)	2
Grade 3 (more aggressive appearance)	3

Applying the formula gives scores that provide the three prognosis groups:

Score less than 3.4	Good prognosis
Score between 3.4–5.4	Moderate prognosis
Score more than 5.4	Least favourable prognosis

Symptoms and signs of breast cancer

History and physical examination

In the first instance, women who find something in their breast that they are concerned about should visit their General Practitioner (GP) to be examined. A referral to the breast clinic of a breast specialist will be made if the GP feels that it is necessary to have further assessment. In the UK, if a breast cancer is suspected, the government guidelines require that the woman will normally be sent an appointment for the breast clinic within two weeks after being referred by their GP. At the breast clinic, a medical history is taken with special reference to the woman's complaint. Common reasons for being referred to a breast clinic are:

- Breast lump
- Asymmetry/distortion
- Changes in the skin
- Nipple eczema or scaling
- Nipple inversion (indrawn nipple)
- Nipple discharge
- Breast pain
- Swelling/Inflammation
- Family history of breast cancer or other cancers.

After the medical history is taken, women undergo a physical examination by the breast specialist. This can be a breast surgeon, breast physician or nurse specialist with adequate training or supervision. The examination requires the woman to remove all her clothes above her waist. Women can ask for a chaperone to be in the room while the examination takes place. The breasts are looked at from different angles, and with the woman in the upright position and then leaning forward, and with the arms in different positions. The breasts are then felt for any change in the texture of the breast tissue or the presence of a lump. The areas above the clavicles (collarbones) and axillae (armpits) are also examined.

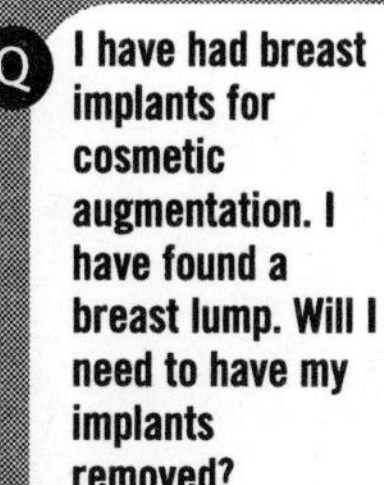

Q I have had breast implants for cosmetic augmentation. I have found a breast lump. Will I need to have my implants removed?

A You will need to have your breast lump checked out by your GP who will refer you to a breast specialist if further investigations are required. You will have a 'triple assessment' if a lump is present. If you need to have a FNA (fine needle aspirate) or a core biopsy, they will usually be done under ultrasound control to reduce the risk of puncturing your breast implant with the needle. Whether you need to have your implant removed or not will depend on what further treatment is necessary. Every woman's case is individual. Tell your doctors what your preferences are and ask what options are available to you.

Breast lump

A lump is the most common way that a breast cancer presents itself. However, most breast lumps are benign, especially those found in young women. Most women find a lump in their breast themselves. Triple assessment is used for a lump in the breast. Triple assessment involves a clinical examination, imaging (using mammography and/or breast ultrasound) and a tissue diagnosis (see Chapter 3, page 53).

myth
Cancerous lumps are often painful.

fact
Most cancerous lumps are painless.

Breast cancer lump

Typical cancerous lumps feel hard and have an indistinct surface or border. They gradually increase in size over time. They can cause puckering or dimpling of the overlying skin. Most are painless. They can be stuck down to the chest wall or ulcerate through the skin.

Benign breast lumps

Benign lumps are usually smooth and mobile (move easily beneath the skin). They can be tender or painless. The most common cause of a benign lump is a cyst or a fibroadenoma.

Cyst

Cysts are fluid filled lumps and they feel smooth and mobile. They can sometimes feel quite hard, cause pain and be tender. Cysts are benign almost all of the time. Benign breast cysts do not usually need to be surgically removed. If they are large, they may require aspiration (the fluid is drawn out with a needle), sometimes repeatedly. If very troublesome (painful and requiring frequent aspiration), surgical removal may be worthwhile. Typical cyst fluid does not need to be sent for **cytological examination**. Typical cyst fluid can be green, brown or straw coloured. If it

cytological examination
Examination (by a specialist doctor) of cells under the microscope in order to make a diagnosis.

is blood stained, it should be sent for cytological examination as it could be related to a growth that could be benign or malignant. If a cyst can still be felt after it has been aspirated, it is usually treated like a lump and investigated like one with 'triple assessment'.

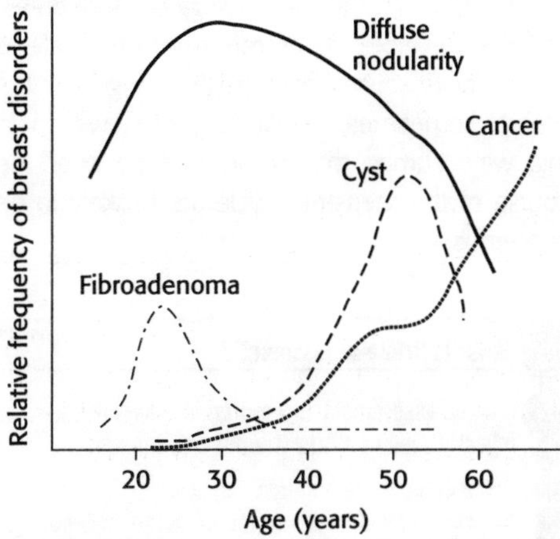

Figure 4 Types of lumps versus age.
Source: Copyright NHS Breast Screening Programme, reproduced with permission.

Fibroadenoma

Fibroadenomas are benign solid lumps that arise from breast lobules, found usually in women between 15–25 years of age. In older women they occur less frequently. Fibroadenomas are usually mobile, painless, spherical and have smooth margins. They are generally single and not larger than 2 cm in diameter. Uncommonly, they can be multiple or larger than 5 cm in diameter, and then they are considered to be abnormal. Triple assessment is usually necessary to ensure that it is a benign lump. When small, no treatment is necessary. Large fibroadenomas that cause breast distortion or are obvious can be surgically removed. Most fibroadenomas remain

myth
All fibroadenomas should be surgically removed.

fact
A fibroadenoma is a benign breast lump. About two-thirds of them remain the same size or become smaller with time. Surgical removal is only necessary if the fibroadenoma is very large or obvious or causes discomfort or distortion.

the same size or become smaller with age. One-third will increase in size, especially during pregnancy.

Localized nodularity

This is a constant area of lumpiness in the breast and, if it is persistent, it is investigated like a breast lump with triple assessment. Most localized nodularity is caused by benign changes in the breast. Sometimes, breast cancer shows up in this way. Lumps that come and go over the course of the menstrual cycle are unlikely to be cancerous.

Q **What is 'triple assessment'?**

A A triple assessment is a systematic method of investigation of a breast lump and consists of:

- a clinical examination
- radiological imaging (mammogram or breast ultrasound)
- tissue diagnosis (usually by fine needle aspirate – FNA – or a core biopsy – see Chapter 3, pages 53 and 54)

Asymmetry

At the time of breast development during adolescence, the breasts can grow at a different rate and be asymmetrical. This is common and is of no concern apart from cosmetically, if **asymmetry** is marked.

asymmetry
Imbalance.

Asymmetry caused by a large lump (for example, a giant fibroadenoma) is very uncommon in Western populations. A breast cancer may cause a newly detected change in the size or shape of a breast in an older woman (see Colour Plate 4). Long-standing asymmetry is not likely to be due to a cancer.

Changes in the skin

Dimpling, puckering, pitting ('peau d'orange' or orange peel appearance), ulceration of the skin or a skin nodule can be a sign of an underlying breast cancer (see Colour Plate 5). Peau d'orange is caused by blockage of the lymphatic drainage of the skin. It is not a common way for a breast cancer to show up, and it usually signifies advanced disease.

Nipple eczema or scaling

An itchy, scaly, red rash of the nipple areola can sometimes be associated with an underlying breast cancer. This condition is called Paget's disease which always starts on the nipple before spreading onto the areola. However, itching of the nipple is more commonly caused by eczema or a fungal infection that normally settles down with an antifungal and steroid cream.

Nipple inversion (indrawn nipple)

An inverted nipple does not necessarily mean the presence of a breast cancer. Many women have inverted nipples that are caused by a number of different reasons. The most common reason is because there is not enough supportive tissue behind the nipple, or the breast ducts are too short so the nipple cannot protrude. Some women have nipples that retract or become indrawn intermittently; these are rarely associated with cancer. The type of nipple inversion that is related to breast cancer is usually unilateral (on one side only, fixed, maybe deviated to one side, becomes more pronounced over time, and is of recent origin in an older woman. (See Colour Plate 7).

myth
Most women with inverted nipples will get breast cancer.

fact
The most common causes of nipple inversion are benign.

Q I have a clear discharge from my nipple. What should I do?

A Whatever type of discharge you experience, go and see your doctor who will be able to discover whether it is normal or abnormal and refer you for tests if appropriate.

Nipple discharge

Discharge from the nipple(s) is common. It can be normal or abnormal. Normal nipple discharge or galactorrhoea is a spontaneous discharge of milk-like fluid as a result of stimulation of the breast. Women on the oral contraceptive pill or who have thyroid disease are more prone to galactorrhoea because of an increase in circulating prolactin hormone levels. It usually arises from multiple ducts and can be from one or both breasts. There is no increased cancer risk. Rarely a prolactinoma (tumour in the pituitary gland) can cause increased levels of prolactin that manifests as nipple discharge. About 70 per cent of women can produce a discharge by squeezing the nipple firmly.

Abnormal nipple discharge can contain blood or be blood free. Bloody discharge can be red or brown (see Colour Plate 8). The most common causes of bloody nipple discharge are intraductal papilloma (usually a benign growth inside the duct), duct ectasia (dilated ducts filled with fluid and benign cells) or less commonly a breast cancer.

Breast pain

Breast pain (mastalgia or mastodynia) is extremely common. Four out of five women experience it at some time in their lives. It can affect one or both breasts, arise from the breast or nearby structures, or be referred pain from elsewhere such as the neck or shoulder.

Cyclical pain

The commonest type of breast pain is called cyclical pain. It usually peaks just before the start of a period and is related to the changes in hormonal levels associated with the menstrual cycle. It can be associated with tender nodular (lumpy) breast tissue that also changes with the menstrual cycle. The best way to determine the type of pain a woman is suffering from is for her to fill in a breast pain chart. This is a type of calendar where the woman records each day whether she has mild, severe or no pain. Women with cyclical breast pain do not usually need any form of treatment once they are reassured that they do not have a breast cancer. Simple measures such as wearing a comfortable supportive bra or not wearing one at all may help.

If the pain interferes with their life, the use of **gammalinoleic acid (GLA)**, the active ingredient in evening primrose oil or starflower oil has been found to be effective in up to 80 per cent of women taking it. For best effect it should be taken at a dose of 360–480 mg GLA each day for at least three months. If GLA does not work, other drugs such as danazol or bromocriptine are available for breast pain, and they have been shown to be of some benefit. Danazol affects the levels of hormones in the body. It has side effects that include weight gain, menstrual irregularities, hair loss and hirsutism (facial hair) among others, and should not be taken if there is a risk of pregnancy. Bromocriptine affects the hormone prolactin that acts on breast tissue. Over half of women with cyclical breast pain respond to bromocriptine. Side effects include nausea, vomiting, dizziness, headache and irritability. A gradual increase in dose will minimize side effects.

gammalinoleic acid (GLA)
The active ingredient in evening primrose oil or starflower oil that helps in the management of breast pain.

Non-cyclical pain

Pain that is unrelated to the menstrual cycle is called non-cyclical pain. This is much less common than cyclical pain. There is often one area in the breast that is painful. A persistent unilateral (one-sided) pain can rarely be related to breast cancer. Most of the time, breast pain is

myth
One-sided breast pain is usually caused by breast cancer.

fact
Most one-sided (unilateral) breast pain is unrelated to breast cancer but it should be checked out as it is sometimes associated with breast cancer.

Tietze's syndrome
Inflammation of the costal cartilage [at the junction between the rib(s) and the breastbone].

anti-inflammatory drug
Drug that reduces inflammation. Common examples are paracetamol or ibuprofen (Nurofen®).

not caused by breast cancer, as most cancerous lumps are painless. Women with non-cyclical breast pain sometimes respond to the measures and treatment used for cyclical breast pain (see above). The best form of management of breast pain is to have a clinical examination, mammogram (for women aged over 35), and to exclude a breast cancer.

Referred pain

The most frequent area for referred pain (pain of non-breast origin) is from the costo-chondral area (the junction between the ribs and the breastbone), and this is called costochondritis or **Tietze's syndrome**. The pain is localized to a very specific spot that is tender. It may become worse on movement or when taking a deep breath. Treatment with **anti-inflammatory drugs** is effective. For severe pain, an injection of local anaesthetic with steroid can help.

Pain can be referred from the neck to the breast. It is usually related to a pinched nerve in the neck and there is often a history of neck injury ('whiplash') or recurrent spinal problems. Less commonly, pain can be referred from around the shoulder. Mondor's disease is inflammation of one of the veins near the breast. It presents as a tender, firm cord. The cause is usually unknown and it usually responds to anti-inflammatories.

Swelling/inflammation

Breast redness, warmth, swelling and tenderness are classic signs of an infection. This is called mastitis. Mastitis is more common after pregnancy and when breastfeeding but can happen at other times. It usually settles down with oral antibiotics and anti-inflammatories. A very rare form of breast cancer called inflammatory breast carcinoma can mimic these signs (see page 26). With this type of cancer, the redness and swelling does not settle down with antibiotics and anti-inflammatories. The diagnosis is made by taking a small biopsy (punch biopsy) of the affected breast skin under a local anaesthetic. A cancerous lump may or may not be felt in the breast.

Family history

It is practical to divide women into three different breast cancer risk groups according to their family history of breast cancer or if there are other cancers in their family:

1 **Low risk** (less than 1 in 6 [17%] lifetime risk of breast cancer)
Women with a history of breast in:

- One first or second degree relative over 40 years of age.

These women should be 'breast aware' and report any changes they are worried about to their GP.

2 **Medium risk** (up to 1 in 3 [30%] lifetime risk of breast cancer)
Women who have the following history should be offered referral to a breast unit:

- a family history of breast cancer:
  - in a relative at a young age
  - in a relative with bilateral breast cancer or ovarian cancer
  - in more members at an older age
  - in a male member of the family
- a family history of breast cancer in only one first-degree or second-degree relative diagnosed with breast cancer over 40 years of age as well as:
  - Jewish ancestry
  - paternal history of breast cancer (two or more relatives on the father's side of the family)

connective tissue
Supporting or framework tissue of the body (for example fat, elastic tissue, cartilage, bone).

- sarcoma (cancer of **connective tissues**) in a relative younger than age 45 years
- glioma (type of brain tumour) or childhood adrenal cortical carcinomas (type of adrenal tumour) in a relative
- complicated patterns of multiple cancers at a young age in a relative.

At the breast unit, each individual woman's risk is assessed and screening is offered according to local guidelines. Annual mammographic screening is recommended for women between age 40–49 years who have a moderate to high risk of breast cancer. For women aged 30–39 years, mammographic screening may be offered as part of research study, as there is not yet enough evidence to say whether it is really helpful or not. From 50 years women should participate in the NHS breast screening programme.

3 **High risk** (more than 1 in 3 [30%] lifetime risk of breast cancer)
Women with a family history of:

- relatives who have had breast and ovarian cancer
- more than one male breast cancer
- Jewish ancestry with relatives who have had breast or ovarian cancer
- relatives with high risk cancer syndromes.

Women should be referred to a breast unit for screening or to a specialist genetics clinic for gene testing. Risk reducing measures should be offered to women if they are found to carry a high-risk faulty breast cancer gene (for example BRCA1, BRCA2 or TP53). Mutations (faults in the gene) of BRCA1 do not increase the risk of breast cancer in men whereas BRCA2 mutations do appear to be a risk factor for men.

Breast awareness

Breast awareness involves being familiar with how a woman's own breasts look and feel. It is a part of general body awareness and of knowing what is normal. It is normal for pre-menopausal women to have tenderness and lumpiness of their breasts in the days before a period because of the effect of hormones on the breast glandular tissue. This still happens if a woman has had a hysterectomy. After the menopause, normal breasts feel soft, less firm and do not usually feel lumpy.

It is useful for each woman to set aside a time every month and to spend a few minutes looking at and feeling her breasts. Things to look out for are:

- Any change in the shape or outline of the breast
- Dimpling or puckering of the skin
- A new and persistent pain or discomfort in one breast that is different from normal
- A lump or thickening, or lumpy area in one breast or axilla (armpit) that is different from the other breast
- A new non-milky nipple discharge
- A change in nipple position (pulled in or pointing in a different direction)
- Rash on or around the nipple
- Bleeding or moist reddish areas on the nipple that persist.

While most changes in a breast are harmless, women should get their breasts checked by their doctor as there is a small chance that the changes could be the first sign of a breast cancer. Women are advised to let their doctor know without delay if they find any change in their breast that is not normal for them.

myth
Bleeding from the nipple is always a sign of breast cancer.

fact
Bloody nipple discharge can sometimes be a sign of breast cancer but this is not usually the case. It is more commonly caused by a papilloma (benign growth) in a breast duct or by duct blockage.

Q **I am pregnant and my breasts are becoming bigger, one more so than the other. What should I do?**

A Many women have breasts that are different in size and when they enlarge during pregnancy, this difference may become more obvious. However, all women should practise breast self-examination during pregnancy and while breastfeeding. Your doctor will examine your breasts early on in the pregnancy. If you find anything new that you are concerned about, you should tell your doctor without delay.

my experience

I fell down and bruised the whole of the left side of my body. I noticed then that my left breast was larger than the right. That happened five weeks before I went to see my doctor. He immediately referred me to the local breast unit. The doctor there examined me, arranged a mammogram, an ultrasound scan of my breast and a core biopsy. It turns out that I have a large cancer in my left breast. I'm not sure if the bruising from my fall alerted me to the swelling of my breast or if it delayed me from going to see my doctor as initially I assumed it was a result of my fall. I am getting treated now anyway.

CHAPTER 3 Tests

Most women who attend a specialist breast clinic with a breast complaint can have their clinical examination and radiological investigations (mammogram and/or breast ultrasound scan) done at the same visit. For women with a diagnosis of breast cancer requiring staging investigations (liver ultrasound, chest x-ray, isotope bone scan or CT scan), another appointment is usually necessary for each test. Screening mammograms are offered to all women after the age of 50, or to women who have a strong family history of breast cancer at a younger age (see page 43).

Breast screening

The UK National Health Service (NHS) Breast Screening Programme provides mammographic screening every three years for all women between 50 and 70 years of age. After the age of 70, women can carry on having screening mammograms on request. When a woman

myth
Older women do not require mammograms.

fact
The older a woman becomes, the higher her risk of breast cancer. Mammograms are a very valuable screening tool for picking up breast cancer, and women over 70 years old can continue with regular screening on request by telephoning their regional breast screening unit.

reaches her fiftieth birthday, she will be called to have a mammogram at one of the mobile or fixed mammography units. The mammogram films are read by two radiologists to check for an abnormality. Women are called back to be assessed in a hospital breast assessment unit if there is a finding on the mammogram that needs further investigation. About 5 per cent of women who have screening mammograms are called back for an assessment. About 1 in 8 women who are called back for assessment turn out to have a breast cancer.

There is no way of predicting who will get breast cancer. Women should be aware of the disease and give themselves the best chance of survival by the early detection provided by mammographic screening. The UK NHS Breast Screening Programme is recognized as one of the most effective breast screening programmes in the world.

my experience

After having had my regular three-yearly mammogram in the mobile van, I received a letter and an appointment for assessment at the breast screening unit. I was petrified. I had never been asked to go back before. I felt both breasts repeatedly and couldn't find anything. When I got to the breast screening unit, I had to wait with eight other women who were in the same position as me. As each of them came out of the examination room, I saw them leave either totally relieved or still anxious, having had a biopsy taken and having to return again for the results. There was a lot of tension in the waiting room. When my turn came, I was examined, had an ultrasound scan and was told then and there that all was well and there was nothing to worry about. It was definitely worth the stress of it all.

Mammogram

A mammogram is an X-ray of the breasts. The breast tissue is compressed (squeezed flat) in two positions and X-ray pictures are taken in each position. Some women may find this uncomfortable and even painful, especially just before a period. Compression is essential in order to give the best picture. Extra pictures are occasionally required to look at certain areas in more detail.

Q What is the radiation risk of having a mammogram? Can I get a cancer from having too many mammograms?

A If you are over the age of 35, you are at a very minimal risk from the small amount of radiation used during mammography. Modern mammography machines use very little radiation, and the amount of radiation you are exposed to is about the same as the dose a person receives by flying from London to Australia and back two to three times; the dose depends on the altitude and length of the flight. The risk of such a low dose is far outweighed by the benefits of early detection of breast cancer.

myth
Women with breast implants should not have mammograms.

fact
Mammograms are not as accurate for women with implants although they still provide useful information. Ultrasound or MRI can be used in addition to mammography for women who have a particular symptom or sign. Women with implants should inform the radiographer that they have implants so that special techniques can be used when taking the X-rays in order to obtain the best views of the breast tissue.

Mammograms are performed in women over the age of 35 years who have breast complaints such as a lump, pain, nipple discharge, nipple retraction or as part of the NHS Breast Screening Programme. Women who have had breast cancer will have mammograms more regularly because they require careful monitoring.

On a mammogram, breast tissue appears white, and fatty tissue looks black. The most common appearance of breast cancer on a mammogram is of a star-shaped (spiculate) area (see Colour Plate 9) which may have some fine bits of chalk (microcalcifications) associated with it, that appear as white specks. It is worth noting that most (80 per cent) of microcalcifications are not worrying as they are usually benign. However, a small proportion can be suggestive of ductal carcinoma in situ (DCIS).

Mammograms are not completely failsafe in excluding a breast cancer. About 10 per cent of breast cancers do not show up on a mammogram and that is why women will sometimes also have an ultrasound scan of their breast(s) or another imaging test such as magnetic resonance imaging (MRI).

radiographer
(for mammography)
Person who operates the X-ray equipment and takes X-rays of the breast.

Q I am 29 years old and went to see the breast specialist with a lump in my breast. I had an examination and an ultrasound but not a mammogram. Why did I not have a mammogram?

A Mammograms are only really helpful for women over the age of 35 years because younger women have more breast glandular tissue. As breast glandular tissue appears white on a mammogram, it can mask diseased tissue that also appears white. This does not easily allow for the differentiation between normal and diseased breast tissue. Mammograms are more difficult to interpret when a woman has very dense breast tissue (Hormone Replacement Therapy – HRT – can cause this), has silicone implants (the implants obscure some of the breast tissue), or if there is scarring from a previous infection or surgery.

Breast ultrasound

A breast ultrasound involves looking at the breasts with a hand-held ultrasound probe after gel is applied to the skin. It is much like looking at the foetus while a woman is pregnant. This is a safe, simple and quick test, and it is painless when the hand-piece is passed over the breast. The hand-piece combines two functions – a transmitter and a receiver. A stream of inaudible, high-frequency sound waves is passed into the breast and the waves bounce off the tissues. The different tissues reflect these sound waves differently and the pattern of reflected waves is transformed into an image using computerized software. An ultrasound is most useful for differentiating between fat, glandular breast tissue, cysts and solid lumps (see Colour Plate 10). Lumps that are smaller than 10 mm (1 cm) may not be seen, and sometimes lumps in fatty breasts can be difficult to see.

Breast ultrasound is used as an additional investigation after mammography and clinical examination for palpable (can be felt) and non-palpable (cannot be felt) abnormalities. It is useful when a mammogram does not give a firm diagnosis. Ultrasound is also used for pregnant women, women who are breastfeeding and those under the age of 35. It is a useful tool to guide the doctor to sample the correct area when taking a tissue sample or when inserting a guide-wire before surgery (see Chapter 4, page 65).

Q **I am pregnant, and I have found a lump in my breast. I am going to see the breast specialist in the breast clinic. What can I expect?**

A Pregnant women are managed in much the same way as non-pregnant women, but do tell your doctor that you are pregnant. You can expect to have 'triple assessment' if there is a clinically detectable lump (see page 38). A mammogram should be avoided if possible in order to decrease the amount of radiation exposure to your unborn child. An ultrasound scan will not harm your baby in any way.

Magnetic Resonance Imaging scan

Magnetic Resonance Imaging (MRI) uses powerful magnetic fields and radio wave signals that are reflected or echoed from the breast.

These signals are measured by the MRI scanner and fed into a computer in order to create images of the breast. This is a painless test and does not involve any X-ray radiation.

multifocal tumour
More than one tumour.

contralateral tumour
Tumour in the opposite breast to the one with breast cancer.

After a physical examination and mammogram have been done, when there is a suspicion of **multifocal** and **contralateral tumours**, and for imaging of scarred and previously irradiated breasts (after radiotherapy), MRI scanning of the breast can be useful as an additional test. It can also be useful for women with breast implants because on a mammogram an abnormality in the breast tissue may be obscured by the implant. Studies are underway to see how effective MRI is for young women at high risk of breast cancer in whom mammography is not accurate because of their dense breast tissue.

The use of breast MRI is limited for several reasons. First, it cannot always distinguish between malignant and benign changes in the breasts. Therefore, more unnecessary biopsies are taken and it is difficult to use MRI for localization and biopsy. Second, it is time-consuming and cannot detect microcalcifications (that sometimes indicate ductal carcinoma in situ) which are reliably detected on a mammogram. Third, patients need to lie very still, face down, in a confined space and it is consequently not suitable for those who suffer with claustrophobia (fear of confined spaces). Fourth, the machine is extremely noisy, and breast MRI scanners are only available in larger centres or research centres.

Methoxy IsoButyl Isonitral or Sesta MIBI scan

Methoxy IsoButyl Isonitral (MIBI) or Sesta MIBI scans are nuclear medicine scans (also called scintimammography) where a radioactive tracer (dye) is injected into a vein, and the gamma camera scanner produces an image of where the radioactivity is taken up. Such scans are used for women who have found a lump, had a mammogram and ultrasound, but where these do not show a clear picture. A breast cancer is more likely to show as a 'hot spot'. The limitations of this test are that it is does not give a clear picture of the location of a cancer within the breast, it is expensive, and takes about one hour to perform. MIBI scans may have a role in women whose mammograms are difficult to interpret (if they have dense breast tissue) or in women who have lumpy breasts where it is difficult to locate a specific lump. They may also be useful in detecting breast cancer that has spread to the axillary nodes. MIBI scans are not widely available because most breast cancers can be diagnosed with more readily available tests.

Tissue diagnosis

When a breast lump or area of concern is found, it is usual to confirm its nature by taking a few cells with a fine needle aspirate (FNA), taking a core needle biopsy (core biopsy) or doing an open biopsy of the lump (surgical biopsy).

Fine needle aspirate

The FNA is a quick test that only takes a few minutes. A fine needle is passed into the lump or area of concern. It is a lot like having a blood test, only the needle is moved around under the skin and passes several times into the lump. A local anaesthetic is sometimes used, but usually the local anaesthetic injection is more uncomfortable than the test itself. The fluid and cells drawn back into the syringe and needle are smeared on to glass slides that are stained with special dyes. A cytopathologist (specialist doctor in tissue and

myth
Having a core biopsy or fine needle aspirate will cause the cancer to spread all over the body

fact
Any needle test is designed to provide a diagnosis and, if a breast cancer is found, treatment can be started. There is no evidence to show that a needle test (or surgery) will cause spread of a breast cancer if the cancer has not already done so.

cell diagnosis) looks at the material on the slides and will normally be able to tell if there are any malignant cells in the lump. The presence of malignant cells gives confirmation of the presence of a breast cancer. It is not possible from this test to tell if the cancer is invasive or non-invasive. A negative result is not considered as accurate for a number of reasons. One of the reasons is that the doctor may not have passed the needle through the tumour. If this happens, it may be necessary to repeat the FNA or do a core biopsy. A core biopsy will tell if a tumour is invasive or non-invasive. This is more helpful when planning surgery as axillary (of the armpit area) surgery is only necessary for invasive cancers.

Core biopsy

A core biopsy is taken with a hand-held device containing a spring-loaded needle that is larger than the one used for FNA. A local anaesthetic injection is placed in the skin; a small cut is then made in order to introduce the needle into the breast. The device usually makes a loud 'click' noise, and it is important for the patient to keep still while the procedure is carried out. Sometimes a core biopsy is done in conjunction with imaging, such as ultrasound or mammography (**stereotactic guidance**), in order to be more certain that the correct area is being biopsied. Some women may find that it is uncomfortable when their breast is compressed using stereotactic X-ray guidance. When using stereotactic guidance to obtain tissue for diagnosis, the woman is seated or positioned lying down with her breast placed in a specially modified mammogram machine. The breast is positioned in a similar way as when mammogram pictures are taken. A local anaesthetic injection is used to numb the area

stereotactic guidance
When an area of concern is seen on a mammogram and it is non-palpable (cannot be felt) and cannot be seen on an ultrasound scan, it can be sampled using X-ray control. This method is called stereotactic guidance and it can be used to pinpoint the exact location of a lesion by using information from mammograms taken from two different angles that is fed into a computer.

before the fine needle aspirate or a core biopsy is performed. A core biopsy is a relatively quick procedure that gives important guidance to ensure that the correct area is biopsied.

The small pieces of tissue taken are stored in a solution of formalin (tissue preservative), sent to the pathology laboratory to be processed, sliced up, stained and then examined under the microscope by a pathologist. The pathologist will look at the architecture of the tissue from the breast lump or area of concern and the types of cells present in order to give a diagnosis.

my experience

The Breast Rapid Diagnostic clinic was all it should have been – fast, professional, polite – but at the same time a truly heart-breaking experience. My mammogram was looked at in my presence by a surgeon and I was informed that I would have to have a needle biopsy. This was done quickly and skilfully by a doctor, assisted by a nurse and watched by a medical student. I was told that I would receive the results the following week.

Vacuum-assisted biopsy (Mammotome or Minimally Invasive Breast Biopsy)

Vacuum-assisted biopsy is a relatively recent method for breast biopsy that relies on ultrasound or stereotactic guidance mammography. It can be used to obtain tissue from non-palpable (cannot be felt) areas of concern that are detected on a mammogram, like microcalcifications (fine bits of chalk), small masses, multifocal (more than one area) and diffuse lesions. A local anaesthetic injection is used to numb the breast and a small cut is made in the skin. Under ultrasound or stereotactic guidance, the operator (radiologist or surgeon) positions the special breast probe into the area of the breast where the abnormality is located. A vacuum line that is attached to the probe provides gentle suction that draws the breast tissue through the opening of the probe into the sampling chamber of the device. The operator captures tissue samples by rotating the sampling device. The tissue samples are processed in the same way as core biopsy samples (see above). With this method, larger cores of tissue are obtained as compared with conventional core biopsies. The advantage of vacuum-assisted biopsy is that more tissue is available for examination, giving a more accurate histological diagnosis. Vacuum-assisted biopsy is not widely used because it requires specialised equipment and expertise, is more time consuming than a core biopsy and is not available in all breast centres.

Surgical biopsy

incision biopsy
Operation involving removal of part of a lump or tissue for diagnosis.

This involves an operation where an incision is made to gain access to the lump, and the lump is removed (excision biopsy), or a small piece of it is taken for histological examination (**incision biopsy**).

Staging investigations

When a breast cancer metastasises, it most commonly spreads to the bones, liver and lungs, and sometimes to the brain. Staging investigations look for any evidence of spread in these areas.

Bone scan

An isotope bone scan (also called a radionuclide scan) involves having an injection of a radioactive fluid (or radionuclide), usually through a vein in the arm, and then having pictures of the whole skeleton taken with a gamma camera machine. The radionuclide travels through the bloodstream and collects in the bones. Most of the radionuclide collects in areas where there is a lot of activity in the bone, and this is detected by the gamma camera. These areas of high activity are called 'hot spots' and they show up areas where there is bone breakdown or repair. Hot spots can signify the presence of bony metastases from breast cancer but they can also be caused by arthritis or other conditions where there is a lot of bony repair and breakdown. The scan is done in the nuclear medicine department of a hospital.

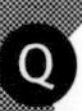

Can a bone scan be dangerous?

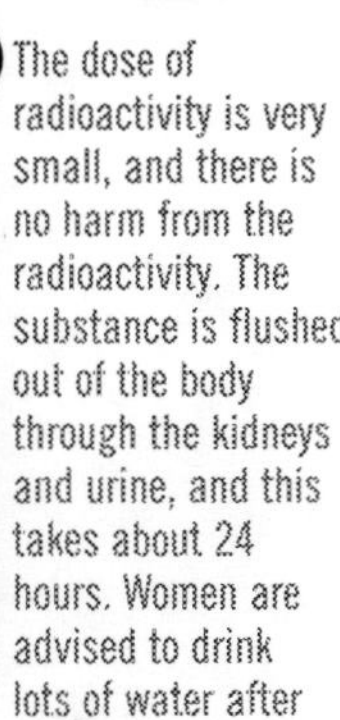

The dose of radioactivity is very small, and there is no harm from the radioactivity. The substance is flushed out of the body through the kidneys and urine, and this takes about 24 hours. Women are advised to drink lots of water after the test.

If there is a chance of a woman being pregnant, there is a risk that the radioactivity may harm the foetus (baby in the womb) and it is advisable not to have a bone scan. Some women having bone scans are advised not to have close contact with pregnant women, young children or babies until 24 hours after the scan, but it is not really known if there is a real risk to them.

Mothers of young babies are advised not to have close contact with or breastfeed their babies for 24 hours after the scan. Women who are breastfeeding their babies are advised to express enough milk beforehand to get their baby through the first six hours after the scan and to get someone else to feed the baby for 24 hours. It is safe for the breastfeeding mother to express more milk for feeds six hours after the scan.

Chest X-ray

An X-ray of the chest will give an indication of whether there is any spread to the lungs or whether there is fluid in the pleural space (between the ribcage and lungs) that may be a sign of spread of the cancer to the lungs. It may also show up metastases in the ribs.

Liver ultrasound

This is the use of high frequency sound waves to provide a picture of the structure of the liver and for evidence of metastases. The ultrasound hand-held probe is passed over the skin after gel has been applied to the skin. It takes a few minutes and is completely painless. Some women may have benign (non-cancerous) tumours or cysts in their liver and it is helpful to know this for comparison later on.

Positron Emission Tomography scan

A Positron Emission Tomography (PET) scan uses the principle that cancers are rapidly growing and so they use more glucose as fuel when compared to normal tissues. PET scanning looks at how much and how fast glucose is used up by a tissue. A breast cancer shows up as an area of increased activity in the breast. PET scanning can also show up metastases in other areas of the body. The main draw back with PET scanning is that it is very expensive, and at present only available in selected centres or research centres where its value is still being studied.

Computerized axial Tomography scan

Computerized axial Tomography (CT) scanning is based on the same principal as an X-ray. When X-rays pass through the body tissues, they are absorbed or weakened at differing levels and so create a 'profile' of different strength X-ray beams once they pass through the tissue. This profile is captured on film and produces the image. Multiple images can be taken at different levels of the body.

CT scanning of the breast would involve too much radiation to be used routinely to pick up a breast cancer. Mammography and ultrasound are safer and give similar information. CT scanning is, good however, at detecting metastases in the liver, lungs, bone or brain.

The results

It is very helpful for women to have someone with them when they get their results for several reasons. It is normal for patients to only remember half (or less than half) of what is said at a consultation; someone else can take notes and ask any questions that may be forgotten. The breast care nurse attached to the breast team is frequently available to answer further questions and to provide a point of contact for the rest of the team. Having someone else there will also provide much needed emotional support.

my experience

When my diagnosis was finally made and mastectomy advised, hysteria, despair, frustration and a loss of control over my life took over . . . I felt that control of my life was in the hands of others. I calmed down soon after and decided to go ahead with the mastectomy and to have an immediate breast reconstruction. Now I am concentrating on healing and getting back to my normal routine.

my experience

Having my husband with me when I went to receive the results of my biopsy was essential. What the patient needs to appreciate is that clinicians are very familiar with the situation and so may not be perturbed by the diagnosis they are giving. On the other hand, the patient can be extremely shocked by the suddenness and seriousness of the situation. From my own experience, I would advise that the patient is accompanied by their partner or someone else who can ask the relevant questions and be there to reassure them.

CHAPTER 4 Treatment

The diagnosis of breast cancer can be a frightening experience. The various treatment options can leave women feeling overwhelmed. This chapter aims to explain what treatments are available for breast cancer and why they are offered. It covers the treatment available to women whose breast cancer falls into these broad groups:

- Non-invasive breast cancer (carcinoma in situ)
- Early breast cancer
- Recurrent cancer
- Advanced breast cancer.

Non-invasive breast cancer

Non-invasive breast cancer (carcinoma in situ) is sometimes called a 'pre-cancerous' disease. Treatment is aimed at local control because the cancer cells are confined to the ducts in the breast. These cancers do not invade the surrounding breast tissue or spread beyond the breast.

There are two conditions termed 'carcinoma in situ' that are very different from each other (see Chapter 2). They are ductal carcinoma in situ (DCIS) and lobular carcinoma in situ (LCIS).

Treatment of DCIS

The aim of treatment for DCIS is local control (the prevention of further spread) using surgery and radiotherapy. This is because, by definition, DCIS is confined to the ducts of the breast and has not invaded the surrounding breast tissue or spread beyond the breast. It is thought to be a pre-invasive cancer because given time, and if left untreated, most will eventually become invasive.

Surgical treatment involves breast conserving surgery or mastectomy. Breast conserving surgery is followed by post-operative **adjuvant radiotherapy**. Some women with very small and low-grade tumours may not need radiotherapy, and this is being studied in clinical trials. Mastectomy for DCIS results in the lowest risk of recurrence. If DCIS recurs after primary therapy, half of recurrences are found to contain an invasive cancer (see page 63).

adjuvant systemic therapy
Therapy such as chemotherapy or hormonal therapy that is given in addition to primary therapy (usually surgery).

Tamoxifen as an adjuvant systemic therapy for DCIS after surgery and radiotherapy has not been found to be of use in reducing local recurrence rates in the treated breast. However, there is evidence to show that tamoxifen reduces the risk of breast cancer arising in the opposite breast.

Management of LCIS

LCIS is considered to be a risk factor for breast cancer rather than a cancer in itself. It very rarely progresses to be an invasive cancer. Careful follow-up with clinical examination and mammography is required for patients found to have LCIS.

Q My surgeon has told me that the lump in my breast is DCIS. This is a non-invasive cancer and it hasn't spread outside of my breast. Why then has he advised me to have a mastectomy?

A Mastectomy is advised if DCIS is widespread and if there is more than one diseased area in the breast. Because it is essential to obtain a clear excision margin (wide margin of healthy tissue) around the tumour, it sometimes involves removing a large amount of breast tissue which might leave a deformed breast. Also, long-term follow-up studies have shown that if DCIS recurs locally, half of these turn out to contain invasive tumours. Radiotherapy is not required after mastectomy for DCIS and chances of local recurrence are minimal after a mastectomy.

Early breast cancer

Invasive breast cancers grow into and invade surrounding tissue, either within the breast or beyond the breast. This is what most people call 'breast cancer'. Invasive tumours in the breast can leave the local area and spread through lymphatic channels or the bloodstream to form metastases (secondary cancers).

One of the first areas in which a breast cancer can be detected when it leaves the breast is the lymph nodes (glands) in the axilla (armpit). Surgery to remove some of the lymph nodes from the axilla will tell whether the cancer has left the breast. When lymph nodes are found to contain cancer cells they are termed 'involved nodes'.

Historically, the first form of treatment for breast cancer was extensive surgery. This was based on the theory that breast cancer spread in an orderly way from the breast through lymphatic channels, and that it could be cleared by aggressive surgery removing the breast, underlying muscles, overlying skin and a large amount of lymphatic tissue from the axilla (Halsted mastectomy). It later became evident that there was no difference in survival rates after extensive surgery compared to less aggressive surgery (Patey or modified radical mastectomy). **Loco-regional recurrences** appeared in half of patients treated either way. Also, chemotherapy was found to help relieve symptoms of patients with advanced breast cancer. These findings led to the theory that some cancer cells which are not clinically detectable may have already left the breast and spread through the bloodstream (**systemic** spread) when the cancer is first diagnosed. These are called '**micrometastases**'.

Modern treatment for breast cancer is therefore aimed at both local and systemic control. Surgery is used to remove the cancer in the breast and any lymph nodes in the axilla that may contain tumour. Removal of lymph nodes from the axilla gives information about the presence and number of lymph nodes involved with tumour and, apart from clearing any cancer in the nodes, is a guide to prognosis and further adjuvant treatment.

Treatment for invasive breast cancer varies according to whether the cancer is found at an early or **advanced** stage. Most breast cancers (90 per cent) are found at a stage where the tumour is confined to the breast. These are called primary operable breast cancers. For these early cancers the two main aims are local control and systemic control:

- **Local control** – to remove the cancer from the breast and any affected lymph nodes from the axilla. This minimizes the chance of the cancer recurring locally (in the area that

loco-regional recurrence
Recurrence of breast cancer in the breast or lymph nodes in the axilla, supraclavicular fossa (area above the collarbone) or internal mammary nodes (behind and beside the breastbone).

systemic
Affecting the whole body.

micrometastases
Microscopic spread of cancer cells to other organs.

advanced breast cancer
The cancer has metastasized (spread) to other parts of the body through the bloodstream or has become very large and spread into the skin or muscles of the chest wall (locally advanced).

metastases
Appearance of cancer in parts of the body outside the original organ. Breast cancer can metastasize to the lungs, liver, bone or brain but rarely to other places.

clear margin
When a cancer is excised, it is sent to be examined under the microscope to ensure that the whole tumour has been removed with a rim of healthy tissue around it. This is to ensure that no tumour is left behind.

breast conserving surgery
Surgery to remove the tumour with a rim of normal surrounding tissue as opposed to mastectomy (removal of the whole breast).

wide local excision or lumpectomy
Surgical removal of the lump with a wide (usually about 1 cm) margin of normal tissue surrounding the tumour.

segmentectomy
Surgical removal of a segment of the breast.

the cancer first appeared). Surgery and adjuvant radiotherapy are used for local control

- **Systemic control** – adjuvant systemic therapy in the form of chemotherapy and hormonal therapy is used to destroy any cancer cells that may have already spread from the breast into the lymphatic system or bloodstream (systemic spread). This is in order to reduce the rate of relapse in other organs (**metastases**).

Local control – surgery

The best way to completely remove an early breast cancer is to surgically excise it with a **clear margin**. Breast cancer surgery may therefore involve removal of part of the breast (breast conserving surgery) or the whole breast (mastectomy).

Breast conserving surgery

The aim of **breast conserving surgery** is to remove the tumour with a clear margin of healthy tissue around it. It is important to have a clear margin because the risk of local recurrence is much higher if some of the tumour is left behind in the breast. Adjuvant radiotherapy is given to the remaining breast tissue to kill any clinically undetectable cancer cells in the breast. This also lowers the risk of local recurrence of the cancer. Clinical trials are being carried out to find out if radiotherapy can be omitted for some women with very small or low-grade tumours where the risk of local recurrence is very small.

Examples of breast conserving surgery include **wide local excision** (see Colour Plate 11a) or **lumpectomy, segmentectomy** and

quadrantectomy (see Figure 5). The amount of breast tissue removed in each procedure is different. The choice depends on the site and size of the tumour within the breast and whether or not there is a large area of the breast involved with DCIS. For large areas of DCIS, a larger margin of tissue around the tumour is removed because of the structure of the ducts within the breast.

quadrantectomy
Surgical removal of a quarter of the breast.

Wire localization

If the cancer is non-palpable (cannot be felt), it may be necessary to mark the location of the tumour with a wire so that the surgeon can follow the wire down to find the tumour within the breast. Before the operation, the tumour is visualized either using ultrasound (ultrasound guidance) or X-rays (stereotactic guidance) and the wire is put into the breast tumour under a local anaesthetic. This is called 'wire localization'.

At operation, the tumour and surrounding rim of normal breast tissue is surgically removed with the wire. An X-ray is taken of the tissue specimen in order to ensure that the correct area has been removed. At the same operation, further tissue can be removed from the cavity in the breast if the X-ray indicates that this is necessary.

The breast surgeon will send all of the tissue removed at operation to be examined by a **histopathologist**. This is to give essential information about the size, grade, hormone receptor and margin status of the tumour, and whether or not there is **lymphovascular invasion** or spread to the lymph nodes. This important information is a guide to whether or not adjuvant treatment will be of benefit, whether or not the tumour has been adequately excised and also gives a forecast of that individual's prognosis.

histopathologist
An expert in the branch of medicine relating to clinical diagnosis of disease using laboratory methods.

lymphovascular invasion
Cancer cells have invaded tiny lymph channels or blood vessels in the tissue surrounding the tumour.

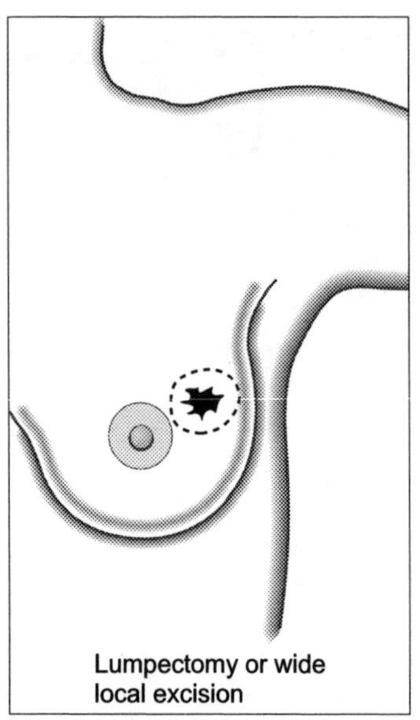

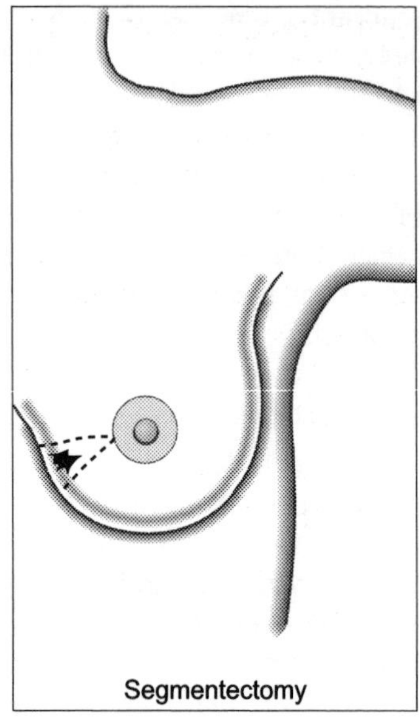

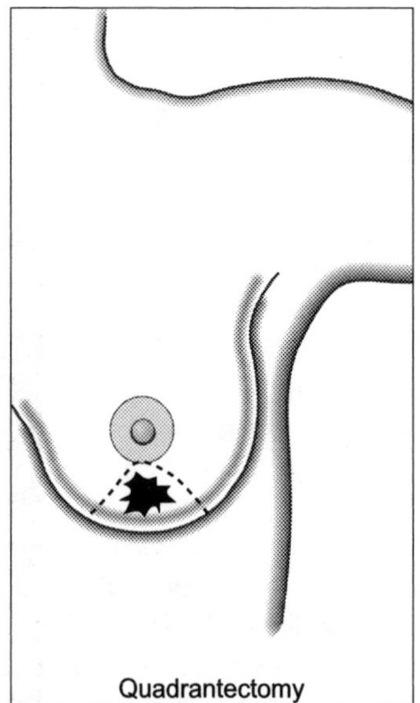

Figure 5 Surgery for primary breast cancer.

Reconstruction after breast conserving surgery

After breast conserving surgery, there may be an obvious defect in the breast such as a contour deformity, poor shape or asymmetry, especially if the tumour is of a large size or in an obvious position. It is best to avoid these defects by reconstruction at the time of tumour excision because they are more difficult to correct later (see page 86).

Mastectomy

Mastectomy involves removal of the whole breast. The aim of a mastectomy is to remove all of the breast tissue so that the risk of local recurrence is reduced. In practice, it is impossible to remove 100 per cent of breast tissue, and in reality a small amount of breast tissue is left behind. Mastectomy is recommended for:

- Large tumours
- Widespread cancer
- Multifocal (more than one tumour in the same breast) disease
- Advanced local disease
- Breast cancer in males
- Recurrent tumours
- A previously irradiated breast
- A tumour located in a position that would leave an unacceptable appearance with partial mastectomy or wide local excision.

Sometimes women prefer to have a mastectomy rather than breast conserving surgery and radiotherapy. The reasons are because they prefer a flat scar rather than what might be a cosmetically deformed breast, or they may not wish to have radiotherapy.

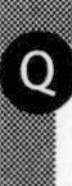

Q I am pregnant and have just been diagnosed with breast cancer. I want to keep my baby. Why do I have to have a mastectomy rather than breast conserving surgery?

A Breast conserving surgery is usually followed by adjuvant radiotherapy to the remaining breast tissue in order to reduce your risk of a local recurrence. Radiotherapy is contraindicated (not advised) during pregnancy because of the potential injury to your foetus.

When mastectomy is combined with removal of lymph nodes from the axilla, it is termed a 'modified radical' or 'Patey' mastectomy. When the pectoralis major or minor muscles are also removed with the breast, the procedure is termed 'radical mastectomy' or 'Halsted mastectomy'. Radical mastectomy is rarely done now. Breast reconstruction is possible for most women having a mastectomy. About half of women who are offered breast reconstruction opt to have it done. Women who are suffering with other illnesses or who need adjuvant radiotherapy may be advised not to have an immediate breast reconstruction but may go on to have a reconstruction at a later time.

myth

If I have a mastectomy rather than breast conserving surgery, I think I will have a better chance of living longer.

fact

Survival rates are similar for women who have a mastectomy compared to those having breast conserving surgery followed by adjuvant radiotherapy, although local recurrence rates may be higher for those women having breast conservation.

A variable amount of breast skin is removed at the time of mastectomy. If an immediate breast reconstruction is done, more skin can be preserved and the skin envelope can be filled immediately. This usually leaves a shorter scar. If an immediate reconstruction is not done, the surgeon removes more breast skin in order to leave a neat flat scar.

Sub-cutaneous or skin sparing mastectomy

nipple–areola complex

The nipple with its surrounding dark pigmented skin.

A sub-cutaneous mastectomy involves removal of the breast tissue where the skin of the breast and the **nipple–areola complex** is preserved. It is possible to do this for women who have a low risk of having a residual tumour in that area, with a non-invasive tumour, and sometimes where the tumour is not close to the nipple. A skin sparing mastectomy involves removal of all of the breast tissue and the nipple-areola complex.

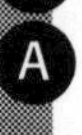

Q What will my scar look like?

A The placement and length of your scar will depend on the site and size of your breast cancer. Ask your surgeon where your scar will be placed and what it is likely to look like in the future.

Q **I have had a lumpectomy but my surgeon recommends a further operation, because my tumour was not completely excised. What does this mean? Why do I need another operation, and can I still keep my breast?**

A Another operation is required because there is a high chance that there is a part of the tumour left behind in your breast. This will put you at a higher risk of the cancer recurring in your breast if a further operation is not done to clear the entire tumour. You may have a large enough breast so that when more tissue is removed, you will have enough breast tissue left behind to give you an acceptable cosmetic result. A mastectomy may be required if there is not enough breast tissue left behind to reshape into a breast that looks acceptable. Bear in mind that should the tumour not be cleared after the second operation, you may then need another operation, which might mean a mastectomy. Also, you will require radiotherapy after breast conserving surgery but you may not if you choose a mastectomy.

Q **I have heard that women do better if they have their operation in the second half of their menstrual cycle. Should I ask for my operation to be done then?**

A This is still an unanswered question. Several retrospective studies have shown that survival is better and recurrence rates are lower if women have their breast cancer excision surgery in the second half (luteal phase) of their menstrual cycle. Other studies have not shown any difference in survival figures or recurrence figures. At present there is not enough evidence to show that we should schedule dates for surgery according to a woman's menstrual cycle. Trials are underway looking for the answer. If you have a choice of dates and it is practical and convenient for you and your surgeon for your surgery to take place in the luteal phase, it would seem the better choice as long as it does not cause unnecessary delay.

myth

Having surgery will make my breast cancer spread around my body.

fact

Surgery is done to remove your breast cancer and will not cause the cancer to spread. Sometimes there are clinically undetectable cancer cells that have already left the breast. Adjuvant systemic therapy is given to 'mop' them up if that is likely.

my experience

I was worried about the lump in my right breast and my daughter encouraged me to have it checked by my GP. My GP got me an appointment at the One Stop Breast Clinic in my local hospital. It turned out to be cancer. I discussed it with the surgeon and we decided to go for a mastectomy as the lump was just next to my nipple. I wanted to be rid of the cancer and didn't mind losing my breast. When I went into hospital, another doctor examined me and persuaded me that I didn't need a mastectomy. He said that I would lose my nipple but that it would be just as good an operation as a mastectomy. I went ahead. When I got the results, they hadn't managed to take it all out. I had to go back for another operation – the mastectomy. I was very relieved to hear that it had been completely removed when I next went back for the results. It is more than seven years since all that happened. I now have four grandchildren and hope to see a few more.

Axillary surgery

One of the first areas that a breast cancer spreads to is the lymph nodes (glands) in the axilla (armpit) or, less commonly, the internal mammary chain (lymph nodes behind the edge of the breastbone). There are about 20–35 lymph nodes under the arm. Removal of some of the lymph nodes from the axilla gives information about whether or not a breast cancer has spread outside the breast. The number of nodes involved with tumour is the single most important predictor of outcome for breast cancer. This information is used to stage the cancer and to guide recommendations for adjuvant treatment. If there is a high likelihood of the lymph nodes being involved with tumour, an axillary lymph node clearance operation will remove the tumour from that area.

Axillary lymph node procedures

A number of different axillary lymph node operations can be done, and the choice depends on the number of nodes that are to be removed. Axillary clearance operations aim to clear most of the lymph nodes in the axilla. 'Axillary sampling' operations aim to remove only a few nodes that are the most likely ones to be involved if the cancer has left the breast. Sampling procedures can be guided using radioactive or blue dye (sentinel node biopsy), or unguided.

Axillary clearance (Levels 1–3)

This operation involves removal of the lymph nodes from the axilla. The number of nodes removed depends on the level of clearance in relation to the pectoralis minor muscle:

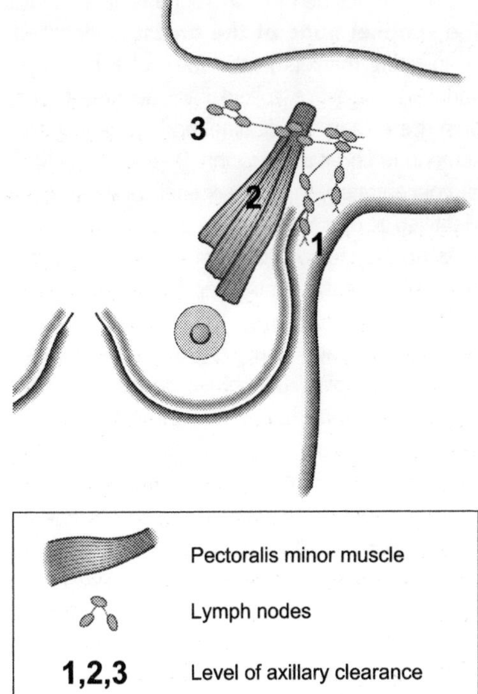

Figure 6 Levels of axillary clearance.

- Level 1 – nodes below pectoralis minor
- Level 2 – nodes below and behind pectoralis minor
- Level 3 – nodes in Levels 1, 2 and those above pectoralis minor.

Axillary clearance is advised:

- When it is evident that there is a spread of tumour to the axillary lymph nodes
- Where it would avoid radiotherapy for patients having a mastectomy
- If the patient prefers it.

Sentinel node biopsy (guided)

The sentinel node is the first node receiving lymphatic drainage from an area or organ. There can sometimes be more than one sentinel node. The **sentinel node of the breast** is identified by injecting markers in the form of a blue dye and/ or radioactive colloid into the breast. The blue dye colours the sentinel node to enable the surgeon to find it at operation. Radioactive colloid is concentrated in the sentinel node and is identified at operation using a gamma probe that picks up the radioactivity from the sentinel node. In most cases the sentinel node is found in the axilla.

sentinel node of the breast
The first node receiving lymphatic drainage from the breast. It is frequently in the lower part of the axilla.

If the sentinel node is found to contain tumour, it implies that other nodes may also contain tumorous tissue. Further treatment will then be necessary. The options are an axillary clearance or radiotherapy to the axilla. The advantage of an operation to clear the axilla is that it gives information on how many nodes contain tumour, and this is a guide to prognosis. The disadvantage is that it involves another general anaesthetic and possible side effects – discomfort and a risk of lymphoedema (swelling of the arm), and a further hospital stay. This must be weighed up against the practicalities and the

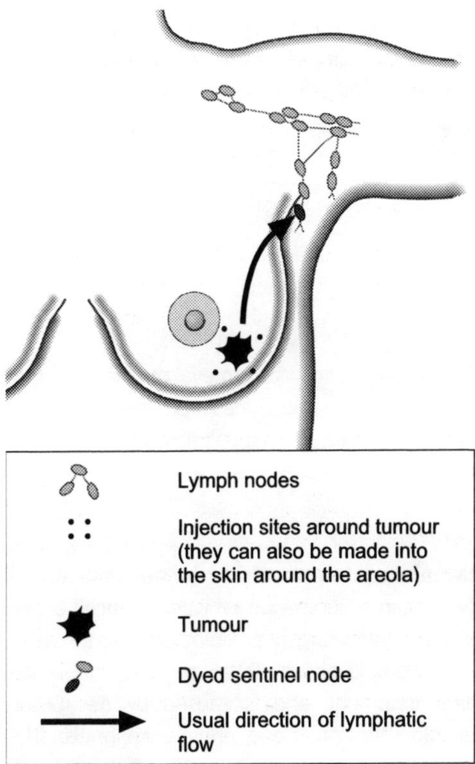

Figure 7 Sentinel node biopsy.

possible side effects involved in having a course of radiotherapy (see pages 74 and 96).

The sentinel node biopsy procedure is a good option for small breast cancers where there is only a small chance of the nodes being involved with tumour. For tumours measuring 2 cm or under there is less than a 40 per cent chance of having involved lymph nodes. For larger tumours where the chances of node involvement are higher, an axillary clearance to remove more nodes in the first instance may be preferable to avoid the likelihood for further surgery or radiotherapy. It is currently undergoing further evaluation in the UK.

Q What are the benefits of having a sentinel node biopsy as opposed to an axillary clearance?

A As only one or two sentinel nodes are removed, there is a minimal risk of surgical complications, and it is a shorter operation and recovery is faster.

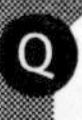

If my sentinel node is found to be free of tumour, does this guarantee that the cancer has not spread outside my breast?

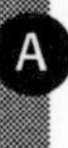

While the likelihood of metastatic spread would be very small with a negative sentinel node, very occasionally spread may already have occurred outside the breast and axilla. Sometimes the sentinel node is not correctly identified (a false negative).

Axillary sampling (unguided)

This operation involves removal of at least four of the largest palpable nodes from the axilla. It is suitable for small or non-palpable breast tumours when the risk of spread to the axilla is small.

Lymphoedema

lymphoedema
Swelling of the arm, breast or chest wall that is caused by an accumulation of lymph in the tissues.

Lymphoedema or swelling of the hand, arm or breast can occur in women with advanced breast cancer or after surgery or radiotherapy to the axilla. It happens in about 10–25 per cent of women after treatment, and is caused by destruction or blockage of the lymphatic channels. The incidence rate varies according to how much surgery is done in the axilla, and lymphoedema is more common when radiotherapy to the axilla is given in addition to surgery. The swelling can range from being mild and hardly noticeable to severe swelling where treatment may be necessary to control symptoms. This could involve wearing compression garments, manual lymphatic drainage (type of massage) or, rarely, surgery. Particular skin care is necessary in order to prevent infection of the fluid-filled tissue.

myth
If I have an axillary clearance, my arm will be swollen for the rest of my life.

fact
No. The chance of you getting lymphoedema is less than 10 per cent with surgery alone, and may be so mild that you won't notice it. If it is more obvious, you might need to wear a compression sleeve and have physical therapy.

Q What can I do to prevent lymphoedema?

A The basic principles behind preventing lymphoedema are:

- Minimizing an overproduction of lymph fluid that is directly related to blood flow. Women are therefore advised to avoid strenuous exercise, excessive sun exposure, excessive heat (for example, saunas, steam rooms or the use of heating pads).
- Encouraging the flow of lymph fluid by avoiding constriction around the arm. It may help to avoid having your blood pressure monitored on the affected arm, not to wear tight clothing or jewellery, not to carry heavy luggage or a handbag on the affected arm, and to avoid extreme cold (for example, an ice-pack).
- Avoiding an infection in the affected arm. The risk of lymphoedema increases with infection because there is an increased blood flow to the area and swelling within the tissue itself may cause blockage of the lymphatic vessels. You are therefore advised to be careful when shaving your armpit and cutting your fingernails. You should use gloves when doing housework and gardening. In addition, the risk of infection may be reduced if you avoid having blood tests or needles put into the affected arm.
- Improve your overall health to encourage good blood flow in healthy blood vessels and provide a healthy immune system to fight infection. Maintaining a balanced healthy diet and doing regular moderate exercise may lessen the risk of lymphoedema. This is because excess body fat is associated with an increased load on the flow of lymph fluid in the lymph and blood vessels and may therefore contribute to lymphoedema. Muscle contraction during moderate exercise promotes the flow of lymph fluid and so lessens the chance of lymphoedema developing. It is best to avoid overstrenuous exercise as it can actually trigger additional fluid production. Consult with your doctor to determine the most beneficial type of exercise for you.

Q What is the lymphatic system and what does it do?

A The lymphatic system is made up of lymphatic vessels, lymph nodes (glands), lymph fluid, lymph tissues and organs (for example, spleen and thymus gland). Excess tissue fluid and proteins are absorbed by lymphatic vessels and transported towards the heart and eventually back into the bloodstream. On the way, the lymph fluid passes through lymph nodes that play an important role in filtering out potentially harmful substances (like cancer cells) and inducing an immune response. This is one of the ways lymph fluid helps the body to fight disease and infection.

my experience

I was delighted when my surgeon said that he could do a sentinel node procedure at the same time as my lumpectomy. It would leave a small scar in my armpit, my recovery would be fast and the chances of lymphoedema would be minimal. After the operation, I was told that I had a positive sentinel node (there was tumour in it) and I would need further treatment. I had two options: either to have an axillary clearance operation or to have radiotherapy to my armpit. I didn't know what to do. I did not like the thought of having cancer left behind in my armpit. Also, I had met a woman who was suffering with chronic pain in her arm and shoulder after radiotherapy to her armpit. It was a really difficult decision to make at the time but, as it happens, I went ahead with the axillary clearance and did not need to have radiotherapy to my armpit after all.

Reconstruction

It is possible to reconstruct the whole breast (after mastectomy) or part of the breast after breast conserving surgery.

Whole breast reconstruction

Breast reconstruction is best viewed as a process rather than a single surgical procedure. It takes several steps to create a breast mound, reconstruct the nipple–areola complex and, if necessary, to adjust the opposite breast for symmetry. Reconstruction of the breast mound can be done at the time of the mastectomy when it is called 'immediate' reconstruction or at a later date as a 'delayed' reconstruction.

The breast mound may be reconstructed using different techniques:

- The use of implants or implant expanders
- The use of a flap (skin and tissue from the back – **latissimus dorsi** or LD flap – abdomen [tummy], buttock, thigh or flank)
- A combination of the above methods.

latissimus dorsi (LD) muscle
Large muscle covering the surface of the back.

Implants and implant expander reconstruction

Implants are made of silicone shells and are filled with silicone gel or saline (salty water). In the past, other fillers such as soya bean oil or hydrogels were used but not found to give satisfactory results in the long term; they have been withdrawn from use in the UK. Expanders are inflatable implants that have a reservoir that can be expanded by the injection of saline through a port that is connected to the implant. The port is placed beneath the skin and gradually inflated over several weeks or months to the desired volume (see Figure 8 and Colour Plate 13).

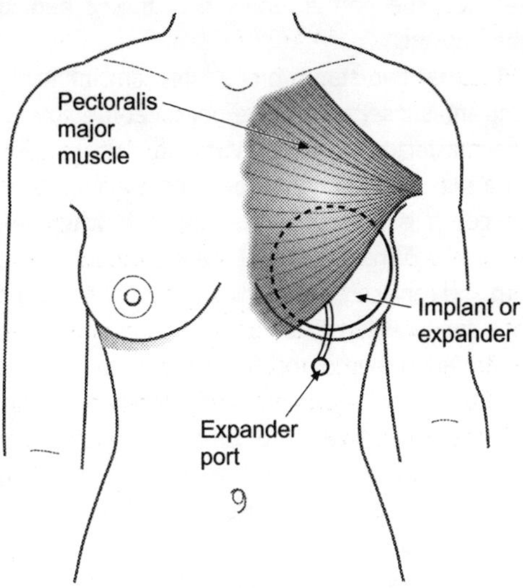

Figure 8 Breast reconstruction using an implant expander.

my experience

Much has been said and written about women's fear of losing their 'femininity' or their partner after a mastectomy, their anxiety concerning their sexual attractiveness, about the irreparable damage done to one's body image, etc. But for me, my fear and abhorrence of mastectomy came from highly personal 'imaginings'. These were war-related images, images of rape and the cutting off of women's breasts, 'medical' experiments in concentration camps – images of brutality and aggression, and not of healing and life-saving procedures. I felt that anything was better than waking up after the operation – mutilated! … I went ahead with an immediate reconstruction but I know that some women are happy not to have a reconstruction.

One-stage and two-stage expander reconstruction

Expander reconstruction can be done in one or two stages. For the single-stage procedure, the inflatable implant that is used has a silicone gel layer around the inflatable pocket. It is the inflatable pocket that is filled with saline (salty water) in stages. When the desired volume is reached, the port is removed or tucked behind the implant.

In the two-stage procedure, an inflatable implant is inserted into the pocket at the time of the mastectomy. The inflatable implant consists of a silicone shell but it does not contain a layer of gel. It is inflated with saline and when the desired volume is reached, the expander is taken out and replaced with a silicone gel filled implant of a similar volume.

The advantage of the single-stage procedure is that a second procedure is not always necessary in order to change the prosthesis. The argument for the two-stage procedure is that it gives an opportunity to make adjustments to the implant pocket in order to give better symmetry once the natural breast skin has settled down and established a stable blood supply.

Advantages:

- Simplest method for reconstruction of a breast mound
- Operative time is relatively short
- No **donor site** scar or potential for complications from the donor site.

donor site
Area from where tissue (for example skin, fat or a flap) is taken.

Disadvantages:

- Cosmetic results are not as good as when a flap is used, especially in the long term.
- Capsular contracture happens in at least 1 in 10 women. The capsule that normally forms around the implant can become hard, painful and distort the breast. A further operation may be required to remove or release the capsule.
- Risk of infection around an implant. It is usually necessary to remove the infected implant and that means a further operation. The cavity is washed out and antibiotics are given. Another implant can be reinserted a few months later when the infection has cleared completely.
- Further operation in the future. Long-term results of symmetry between the breasts are not maintained because the implant tends to stay in the same position on the chest wall while the natural breast changes naturally with age and body weight fluctuations. How long an implant will last is not known for sure. Modern implants should last over 10–15 years.

Flap reconstruction

The use of the body's own tissue for breast reconstruction in the form of a **flap** provides a good, long lasting result. The reconstructed breast feels soft and warm and will change with time and body weight changes. One of the most commonly used flaps for breast reconstruction is

flap
A portion of tissue that is moved (while still maintaining its blood supply) from one part of the body to another.

the latissimus dorsi (LD) flap. It is a reliable and robust flap. Another area from which tissue is obtained is the abdomen. There are different ways in which tissue from the abdomen can be transferred to create a breast (see page 82).

Latissimus dorsi flap

The LD flap can be used with or without an implant or expander. It involves moving the LD muscle, with or without overlying fat or skin, from the back to the front of the chest while still attached to its blood supply (see Figure 9 and Colour Plate 12 as well as Colour Plate 6 and 14).

Advantages:

- It provides a better cosmetic result than the use of an implant or expander alone
- It can provide skin replacement
- It provides a cushion of tissue between the implant and breast skin
- No risk of capsular contracture or loss of the implant with infection if used without an implant.

Disadvantages:

- There is a donor scar on the back – the length of the scar depends on how much breast skin needs to be replaced after the mastectomy
- Longer operative time as compared with using an implant-only procedure, with potentially more complications.

It may be preferable to use a flap without an implant if the flap is big enough, to avoid the possible complications of capsular contracture and infection associated with an implant. The LD flap by itself (without the use of an implant or expander) usually provides sufficient volume and is big enough for women with small to medium-sized breasts, but an operation to the opposite

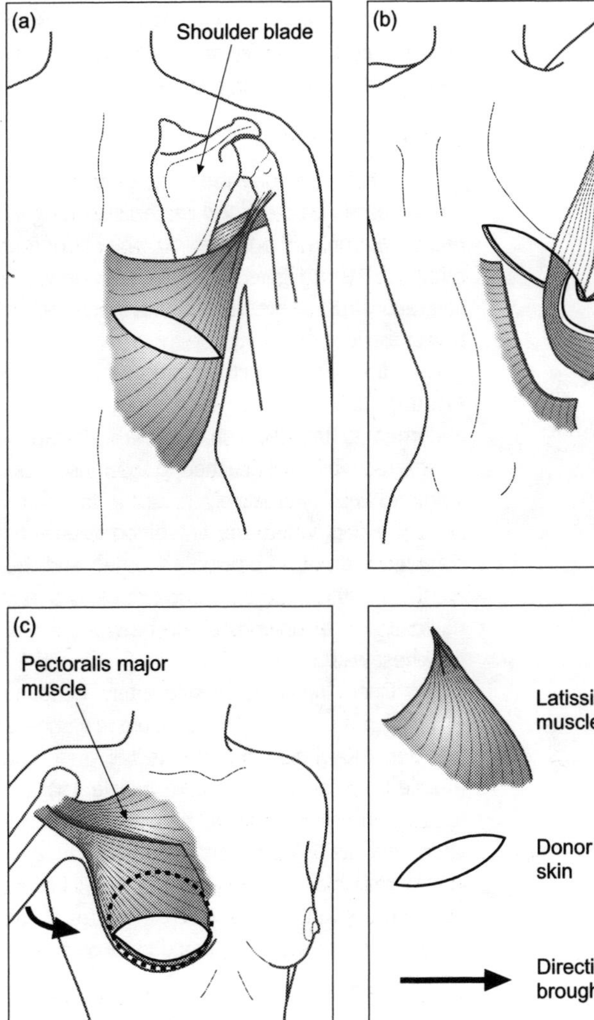

Figure 9 Breast reconstruction with latissimus dorsi flap.

breast (uplift or breast reduction) is sometimes needed to achieve a balanced result. For women with larger breasts, an abdominal flap usually provides enough tissue to reconstruct a breast mound without requiring an implant.

Abdominal flaps

Abdominal flaps involve the transfer of skin, fat or muscle based on the blood vessels supplying the rectus abdominis muscle on the abdomen (stomach) (see Figure 10). They provide warm, soft reconstructed breasts that move and feel like breast tissue.

The transverse rectus abdominis muscle (TRAM) flap can be transferred from the abdomen to the chest in two ways. It can be transferred while still attached to the muscle as a 'pedicled flap'. Alternatively, it can be transferred as a 'free flap' where the tiny blood vessels are completely divided from the abdomen and they are then resutured to a new source using special microsurgical techniques at the new position on the chest wall.

The Deep Inferior Epigastric artery Perforator (DIEP) flap is based on the same blood vessels as the free TRAM flap but the rectus abdominis muscle is left behind (see Colour Plate 15). This reduces the risk of hernia or weakness of the abdominal wall. A sufficient amount of tissue is usually available to create a breast mound without using an implant. Long-term cosmetic results are generally much better compared to reconstruction with implants.

Advantages:

- Provides a better cosmetic result than the use of an implant or expander alone
- Can provide skin replacement
- Provides tissue that is soft and warm and feels most like breast tissue compared to other types of reconstruction

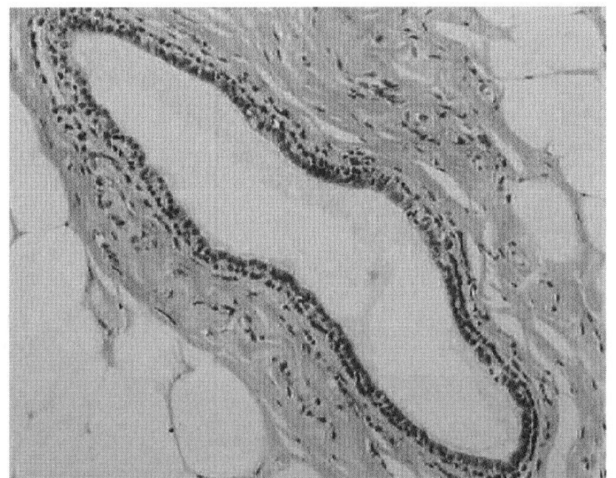

Colour Plate 1
Normal breast tissue – appearance under the microscope. Cross section of a duct lined by normal ductal cells.

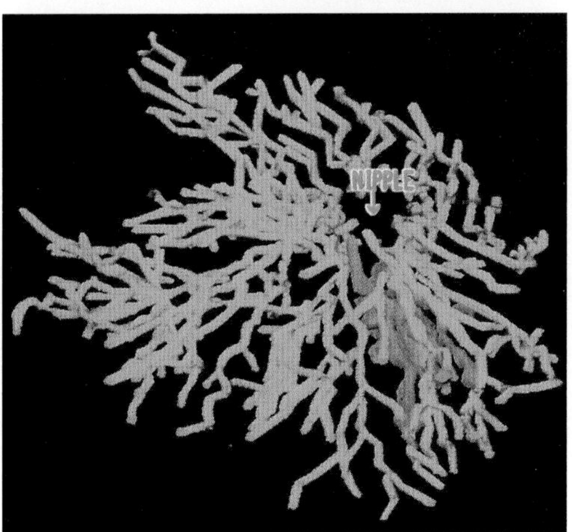

Colour Plate 2
Ductal carcinoma in situ (DCIS is shown in red and the normal ducts are shown in yellow).

CANCER, Vol. 91, No. 12, 2001, pp. 2263–72.

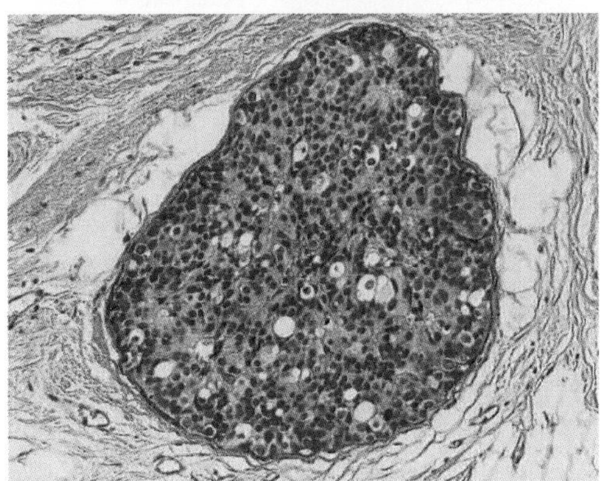

Colour Plate 3
Ductal carcinoma in situ – appearance under the microscope. Cross section of a duct filled with abnormal ductal cells.

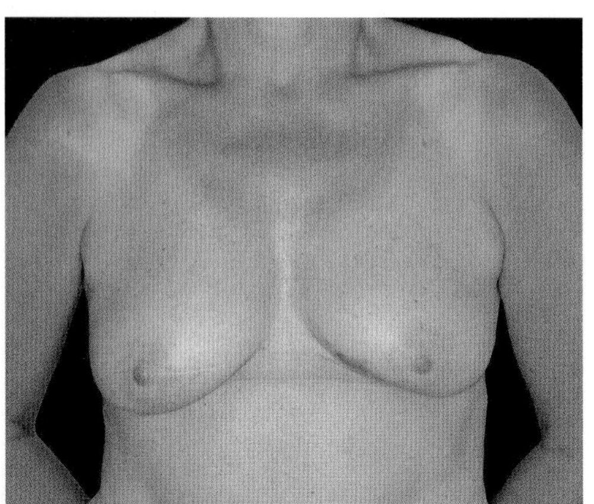

Colour Plate 4
Left breast cancer showing breast asymmetry.

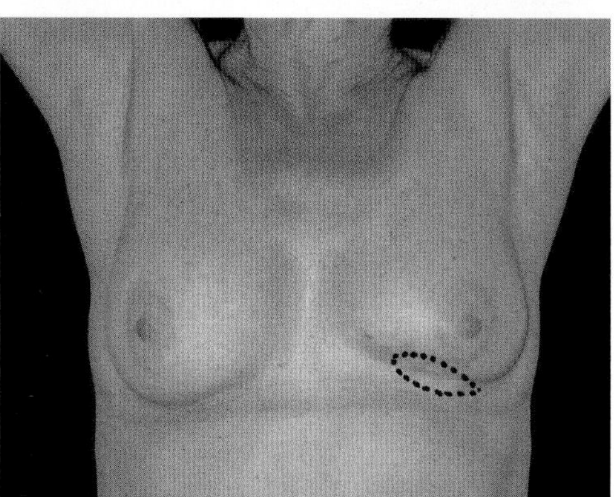

Colour Plate 5
Left breast cancer showing skin puckering beneath left breast when arms are raised. (Same patient as in Colour Plate 4.)

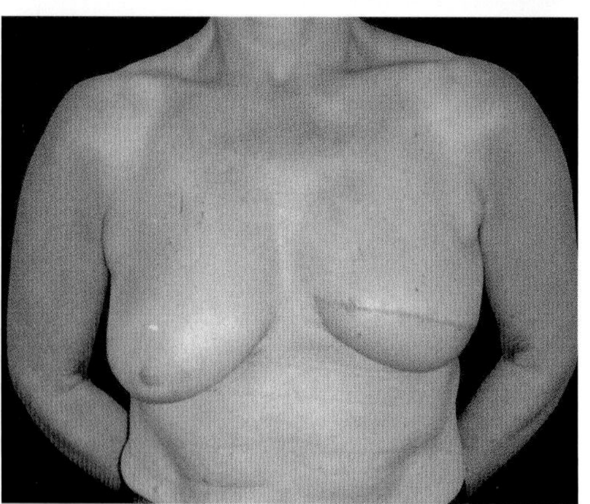

Colour Plate 6
Immediate partial breast reconstruction with latissimus dorsi flap after left hemi-mastectomy (volume replacement oncoplastic technique). (Same patient as in Colour Plates 4 and 5.)

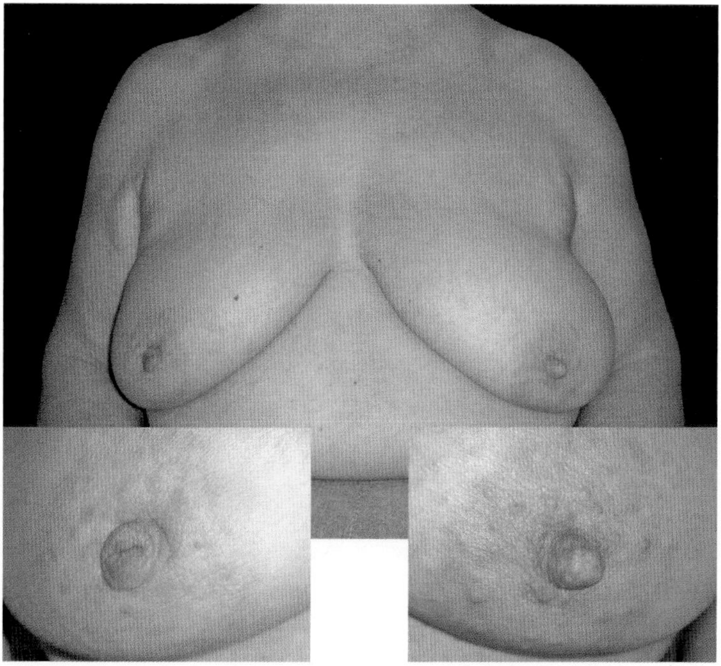

Colour Plate 7
Inversion/retraction of right nipple (associated in this case with right breast cancer).

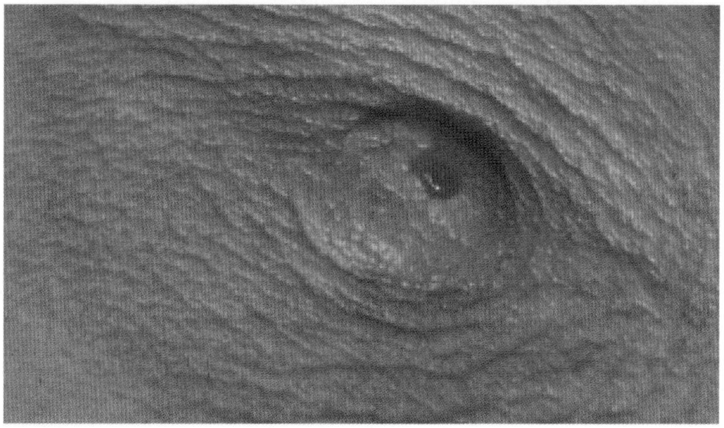

Colour Plate 8
Blood stained nipple discharge (associated in this case with ductal carcinoma in-situ and microinvasion).

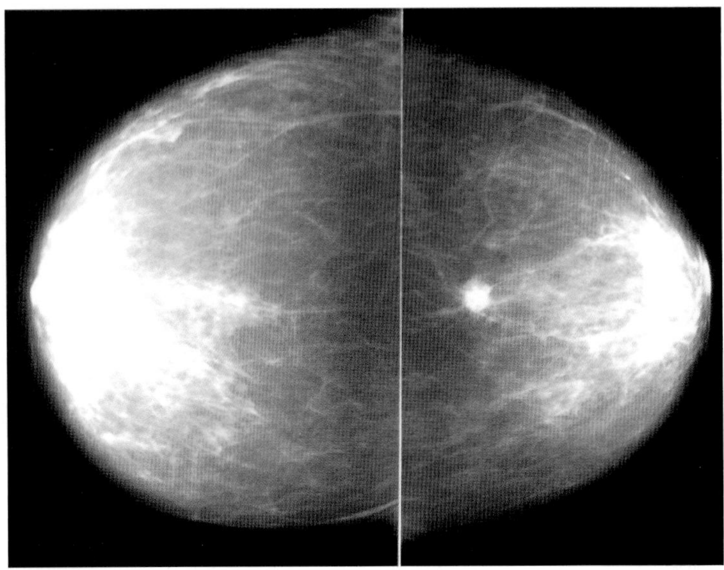

Colour Plate 9
Mammographic appearance of a spiculate mass. In this case showing left breast cancer.

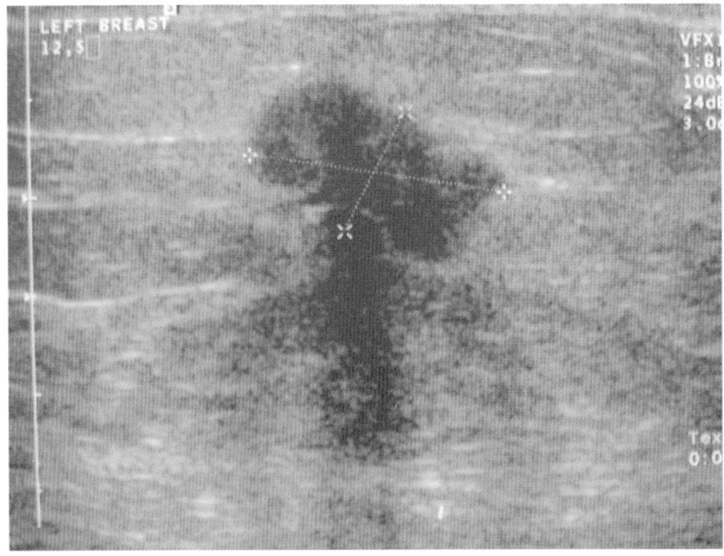

Colour Plate 10
Ultrasound appearance of an irregular solid mass. In this case showing left breast cancer.

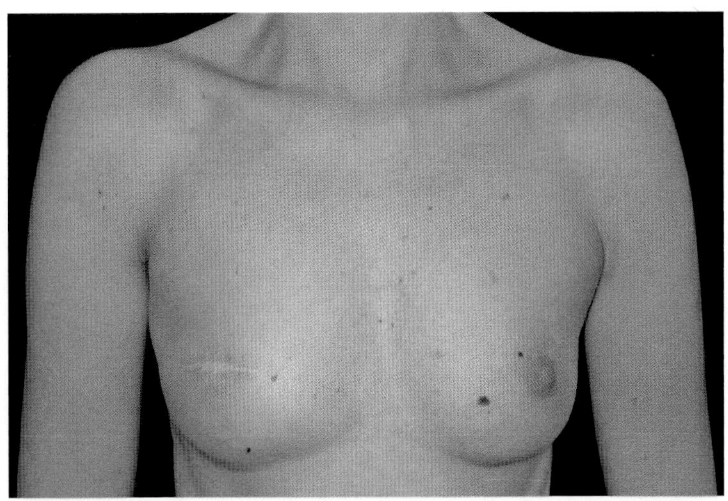

Colour Plate 11a
Breast conserving surgery (central wide local excision) and radiotherapy for right breast cancer.

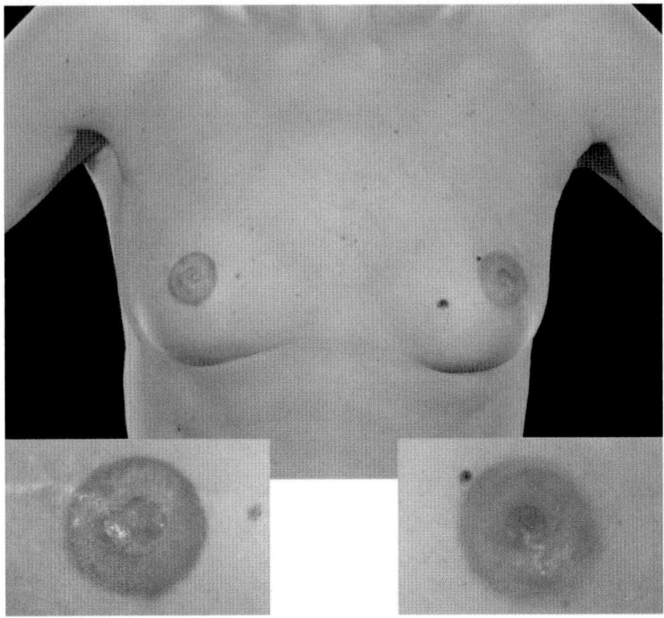

Colour Plate 11b
After right nipple-areola reconstruction with nipple share and tattoo technique.

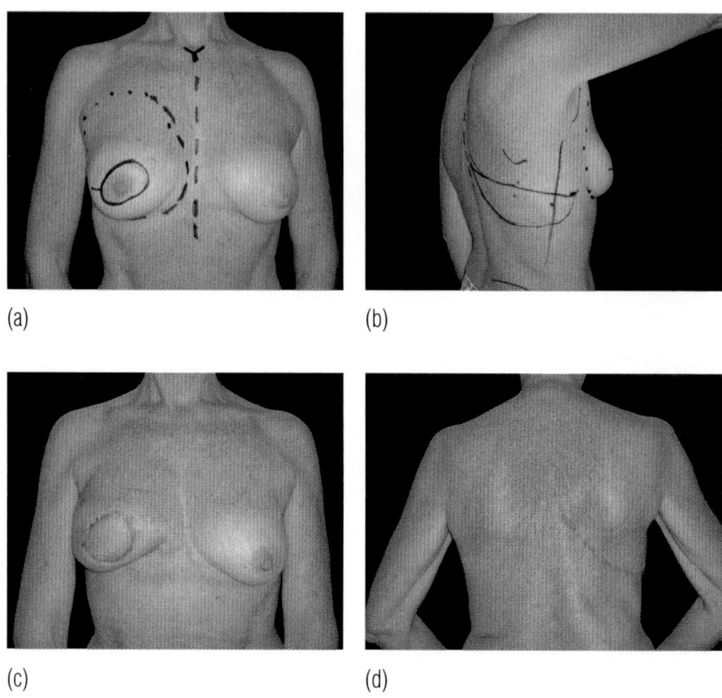

(a) (b) (c) (d)

Colour Plate 12
Immediate breast reconstruction with latissimus dorsi flap following right skin-sparing mastectomy.
(a) Preoperative appearance – the dotted lines show mid-line and extent of breast tissue to be excised, continuous lines are incision lines.
(b) Skin marks showing plan for latissimus dorsi flap.
(c) Three weeks after surgery – nipple-areola skin replaced by skin from back.
(d) Three weeks after surgery – latissimus dorsi donor scar on the back.

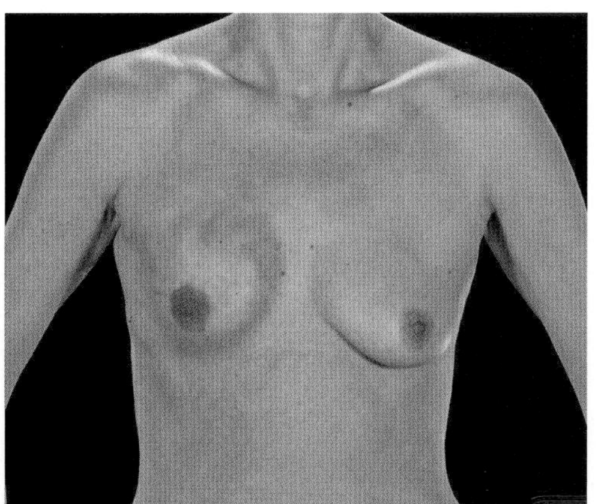

Colour Plate 13
Immediate breast reconstruction with implant expander and prosthetic nipple-areola complex following right mastectomy.

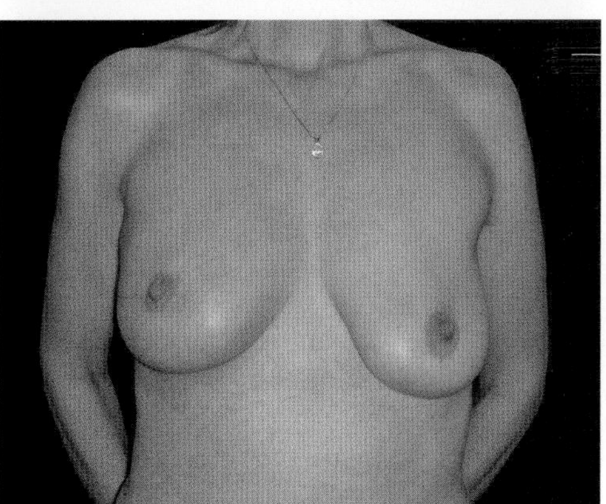

Colour Plate 14
Immediate partial breast reconstruction with latissimus dorsi flap after right upper hemi-mastectomy (volume replacement oncoplastic technique).

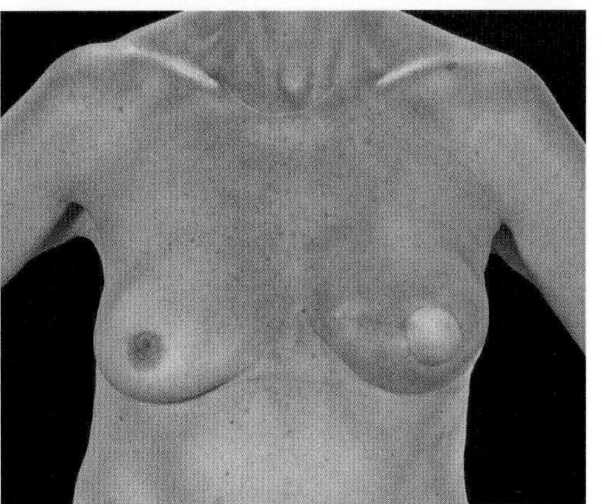

Colour Plate 15
Immediate breast reconstruction with free abdominal deep inferior epigastric artery perforator (DIEP) flap after left mastectomy.

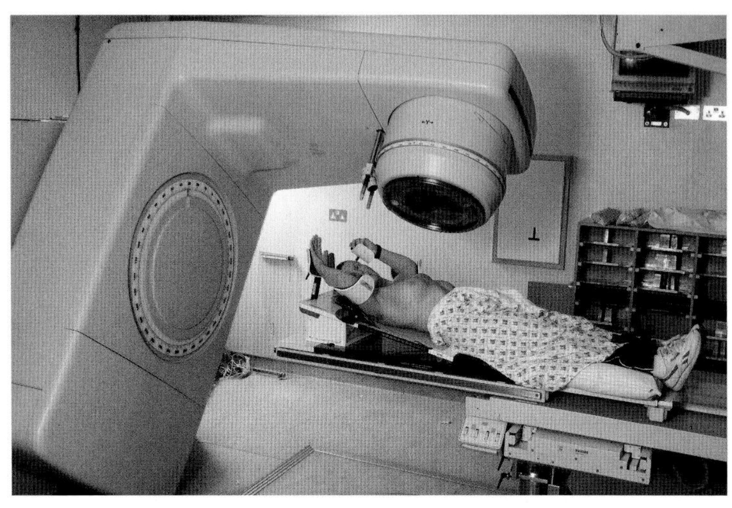

Colour Plate 16
A patient receiving external beam radiotherapy after breast conserving surgery for breast cancer.

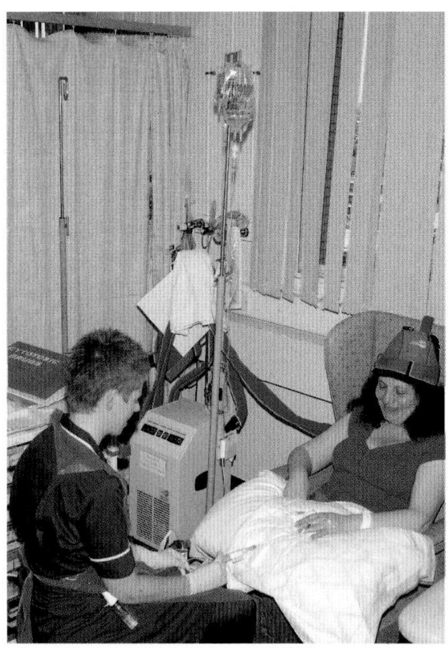

Colour Plate 17
A patient receiving chemotherapy following surgery for breast cancer.

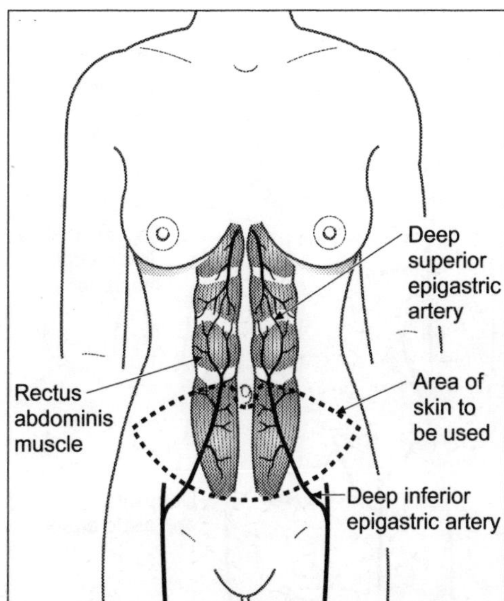

(a) Tissue used for abdominal flap breast reconstruction.

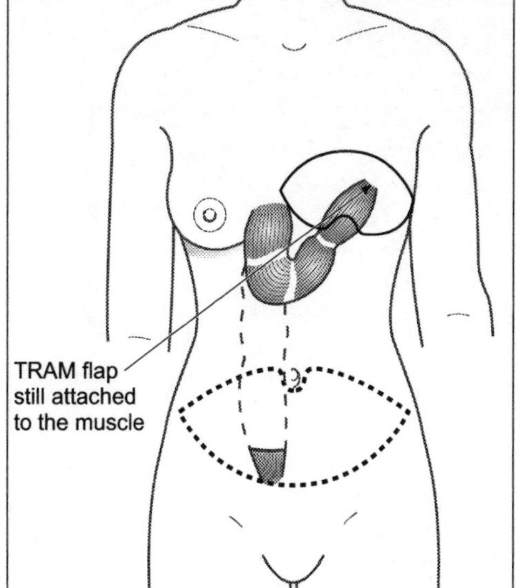

(b) Reconstruction with pedicled TRAM flap.

Figure 10 Breast reconstruction with abdominal flap (a–d).

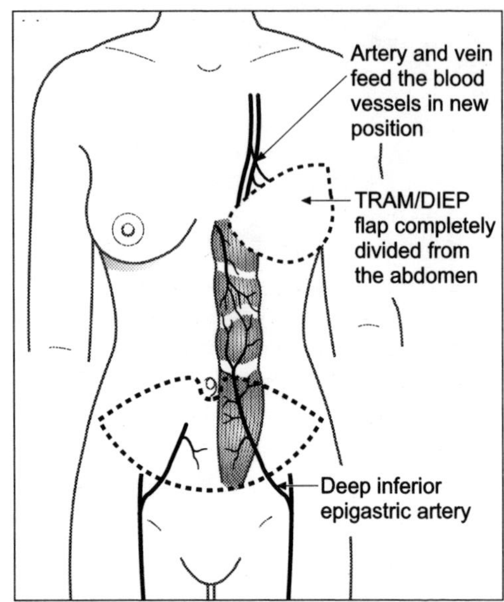

(c) Reconstruction with free TRAM/DIEP flap.

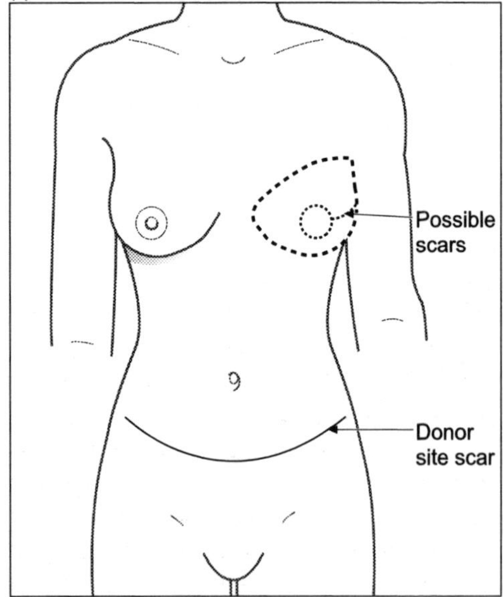

(d) Result with abdominal flap.

- No risk of capsular contracture or loss of the implant with infection.

Disadvantages:

- Donor scar on the abdomen – it looks like the scar from an abdominoplasty (tummy tuck) operation
- Lengthy procedure requiring specialist skills – not all surgeons are trained to perform this procedure and another team may need to be found to take part in the operation
- Risk of flap loss – the flap may die off because of a poor blood supply.

Other flaps

Flaps from the thigh, buttock or flank are free flaps and are not commonly used. These involve highly specialized procedures with a higher risk of failure than the other available methods. Donor site scars are considerable and operative times lengthy. They are only usually offered when the other methods are unsuitable or have failed.

The nipple–areola complex

A prosthetic nipple-areola can be obtained off the shelf or can be custom-made to match the opposite side. The prosthesis is stuck on to the reconstructed breast mound using a skin adhesive. Alternatively, the nipple–areola complex can be reconstructed when the desired shape and size of the breast mound has been achieved. Local flaps of skin or a portion of the opposite nipple can be used to create the new nipple. For colouring the areola, tattoo pigments or skin grafts are used. Tattooing allows a better colour match as the opposite side can be tattooed as well (see Colour Plate 116). Skin grafts tend to fade over

Q What are the disadvantages of an immediate reconstruction?

A The major disadvantages are:

- It is a big decision to make at a time when you not only have to face the diagnosis of a breast cancer but also the loss of a breast
- The initial operation is a more complex one and will take longer than a mastectomy alone.

time and the scar tissue behind a skin graft does not hold tattoo pigment as well as normal skin.

Q What are the advantages of an immediate reconstruction?

A The main advantages of an immediate reconstruction are:

- You do not have to live with the mastectomy scar
- The number of operations is reduced without significantly prolonging the hospital stay
- The overall time spent in hospital and recovering from the operation is less than having it done as a delayed procedure
- More natural breast skin is left behind with the potential for better sensation and shorter scars.

my experience

When I was told that I would need to have a mastectomy, the first thing I thought was that I could not live being deformed with a flat chest. My surgeon explained that it would be possible to have a breast reconstruction either at the time of the operation (immediate reconstruction) or after the completion of my adjuvant therapy (delayed reconstruction). I found out about all the available options on the internet and read all the booklets I could lay my hands on. I couldn't decide. I didn't want my reconstruction ruined by radiotherapy and there was a high likelihood that I would need it. In the end I had the mastectomy, and am having my chemotherapy. I will need to have radiotherapy after chemo and I can take my time deciding what sort of reconstruction to have and when to have it. I wear an external breast form (prosthesis) in my bra and no one can tell that my breast is missing.

oncoplastic technique
Surgical technique combining both surgical specialities of cancer surgery for excision of the tumour (onco) and plastic surgery (plastic) for reconstruction.

Partial breast reconstruction

Oncoplastic techniques for breast conserving surgery

Corrective surgery using **oncoplastic techniques** can be used to reshape the breast or fill in the defect caused by removal of the cancerous breast tissue. The cosmetic result after surgery depends on how big the tumour is and where the tumour is located within the breast. For large tumours or those located in certain areas of the breast (especially those behind the nipple and in the lower part of the breast), it may be necessary to reshape the breast after removal of the lump. Reshaping can be done by moving nearby tissue into the defect, and adjusting the location of the nipple on the new breast mound. This is a 'volume displacement' oncoplastic technique. This will result in a smaller size of breast with a normal shape. An operation to the other breast may be required to achieve a balance. If there is insufficient remaining breast tissue after removal of the tumour, a flap can be brought into the defect to make up the missing tissue. An example of this is the latissimus dorsi mini flap and this is called a 'volume replacement' oncoplastic technique. When the tumour is very large or the breast is small, it may be advisable to have a mastectomy and breast reconstruction because there would not be enough tissue left behind to create a cosmetically acceptable breast.

my experience

The lump in the lower part of my left breast turned out to be cancer. I would lose half of my breast to clear the tumour. My options were either to reconstruct the lower half of my breast with the LD flap from my back or to have a mastectomy. There wasn't enough tissue on my back to recreate my whole breast without the use of an implant. I didn't like the thought of an implant so I had 'volume replacement' with the LD flap from my back. I am back to work now after chemotherapy and radiotherapy and no one can see any difference.

myth
A breast reconstruction will compromise the treatment of my breast cancer and affect survival.

fact
Breast reconstruction does not affect treatment, or alter the chances of detecting a recurrent breast cancer, and it does not affect survival rates.

Q What will be the effect of moving the LD muscle from my back? Isn't it an important muscle and won't I miss it?

A Most women who have had the LD flap for breast reconstruction don't notice any difference in the movement or strength of their arm in their day-to-day activities. However, it is not advised if you are a keen golfer, rock climber or skier.

my experience

I was shocked, angry and very upset when I was told that I had breast cancer. I had just recovered from an operation to remove a breast duct for nipple discharge. The doctor was now recommending that I have my breast removed. I couldn't take it all in. The breast care nurse suggested that I have another appointment so that my partner could be with me. It made all the difference having my partner there. He was able to write down what was being said and remind me to ask the questions we had discussed beforehand. The surgeon explained that there was residual cancer in my breast and since my breasts were very small, removing the central part of my breast, including the nipple areola, would leave me with very little breast tissue and that the result would not look good. I had the option of a skin sparing mastectomy with an immediate reconstruction or a simple mastectomy. It would be unlikely for me to need radiotherapy after the operation and the cure rate was high. I felt much better and went ahead with the mastectomy and immediate reconstruction.

The opposite breast

In order to achieve a balance between the breasts, an operation to the opposite breast may be needed. The breast without the cancer may be enlarged (breast augmentation), reduced (breast reduction) or lifted up (mastopexy). These procedures are normally done at the final stage of reconstruction.

Breast augmentation

Breast augmentation is usually done by inserting a silicone implant into a pocket that is created behind the breast gland or pectoralis major muscle. Women should note that mammography is not as accurate in women who have silicone implants. Women with implants should inform their mammographer (person taking the mammogram) that they have implants so that special views can be taken.

Breast reduction

When reducing the size of the breast, the extra tissue that is removed at operation is sent for examination by a pathologist to check for the presence of a clinically undetectable breast cancer. The incidence of finding a cancer in breast tissue removed for cosmetic breast reduction operations is about 1 in 100. The scars within the breast that result from the reduction operation do not usually cause any difficulties in interpreting a mammogram.

Mastopexy

Mastopexy (breast uplift) involves the removal of excess breast skin, and refashioning the breast tissue to give an uplifted appearance.

Prophylactic mastectomy

Prophylactic mastectomy involves removal of the breast with the intention of preventing a breast cancer from arising. This may be suitable when there is a high risk of developing breast cancer in the opposite breast in a woman already diagnosed with breast cancer; or in women who have a gene that predisposes breast cancer. It is usually possible to do a sub-cutaneous mastectomy and preserve the nipple areola and to reconstruct the breast immediately.

A mastectomy will not remove all of the breast tissue and, while it will reduce the risk of breast cancer, it will not completely eradicate it. It is important for women considering prophylactic mastectomy to understand their own individual risk of breast cancer and to weigh it against the outcomes and risks of having surgery as opposed to close surveillance or taking hormonal therapy as part of a clinical trial.

When a faulty breast cancer gene has not yet been identified in a woman who has a very strong family history, it is important to realize that she has a 50 per cent chance of inheriting the gene if it is found on subsequent testing of another family member. Genetic tests currently on offer only detect about 20 per cent of inherited breast cancers. Better tests are being developed all the time.

A consultation with a clinical geneticist is advisable to calculate each woman's individual risk of breast cancer before any risk-reducing surgery is contemplated.

Complications of surgery

While complications are not common, it is helpful to have an idea of the possible undesired effects of any treatment. Complications of breast surgery are usually not serious if recognized at an early stage and when prompt treatment is started.

General complications

Infection

Infection is uncommon in breast surgery. Redness, warmth, increasing pain or fever can be signs of an infection. Treatment may involve antibiotics, dressings or surgical wash-out of the infected area.

Bleeding

Small amounts of blood that collect in the operated area can be drained away if a drainage tube has been inserted. If blood collects beneath the skin, it coagulates (solidifies) to form a haematoma (see below).

Haematoma

A small haematoma (collection of blood beneath the skin) may resolve itself without further treatment. A large haematoma can cause pressure on the skin, and the collected blood may have to be washed out at another operation.

Seroma

It is normal to have small amounts of fluid that collect beneath the skin – these are called 'seromas'. Drains (if used) carry away this fluid. After the drain is removed, any collection of fluid can be aspirated (drawn out) using a syringe and needle.

Scars

Scars usually take a few months to settle down. They can start off being lumpy. Hypertrophic scars are those that are red and lumpy and take a long time to settle down. Keloid scars are uncommon; they can grow beyond the operated area, are thick and can be itchy.

Contour deformity

After breast conserving surgery, there may be a concavity (dip in the surface) in the breast. This is because of the loss of the tissue in that area. The degree of the concavity will depend on the size of the tumour and the amount of tissue removed at surgery. Oncoplastic techniques for breast reshaping done at the time of original surgery are helpful in reducing these deformities.

Asymmetry

After removal of the breast cancer with a rim of surrounding normal tissue, there is a smaller volume of breast tissue left behind. The degree of imbalance will depend on the original breast size and the size of the tumour.

Wound dehiscence

If there is a lot of tension in the skin, the wound can split apart. This is called 'dehiscence'. It may be necessary to have another operation to repair the dehiscence.

Deep Venous Thrombosis

This occurs when clots form in the veins behind the leg(s) or higher up. It happens when a patient is immobile for a long period of time, for example on the operating table or spending a long time in bed. The leg becomes swollen and may become painful and red. Treatment is by anti-coagulant drugs.

Pulmonary embolus

This is a clot that lodges in the blood vessels in the lung. The clot usually forms in the deep veins of the leg or pelvis, breaks away from the original site of formation and travels into the blood vessels in the lungs. It is a rare but serious condition.

Skin necrosis

If the blood supply to the skin is disrupted, it can die. This is called necrosis. Some causes of a poor blood supply are pressure on the skin, for example a haematoma or a tight dressing. It is more common in smokers.

Nipple–sensory loss or change

The sensation to the nipple can be reduced, heightened or lost if the nerves to the nipple are damaged or stretched during surgery. This may be unavoidable if the cancer is close to or involving these nerves.

Nipple–areola loss

This can happen if the blood supply to the nipple–areola complex is disrupted while removing the cancer or if the nipple–areola has to be moved a long distance when reshaping the breast. A further operation may be required or the area may require repeated dressings.

Fat necrosis (death of fatty tissue)

This can happen when the blood supply to that part of the breast is reduced or cut off when the cancer is removed or when the remaining tissue is moved into the defect. It may cause prolonged wound healing (see below) and a further operation may be required.

Prolonged wound healing

Healing can take a long time if there is an infection, a haematoma, fat necrosis or wound dehiscence. Other causes can be:

- Prolonged ill health or the presence of other illnesses
- Poor diet
- Certain drugs.

Repeated dressings are often necessary.

Complications associated with implant surgery

There are specific risks with the use of breast implants. The most troublesome are capsular contracture and infection involving the implant.

Infection around an implant

An implant is a large foreign body. If an infection occurs around an implant, removal of the implant is usually necessary before the infection can be successfully treated.

Capsular contracture

The body's natural response to a foreign body is to form a scar around it. This is called a capsule. A capsular contracture occurs when this capsule becomes hard and painful. It happens in about 10 per cent of women who have implants. Another operation may be necessary to remove or release the capsular contracture. The risk of capsular contracture is higher when radiotherapy is given after the implant is inserted.

Implant leak or rupture

It is uncommon for modern-day implants to leak or rupture unless an undue amount of force has been applied to the implant. If there is a leak or rupture, silicone may be pushed into the surrounding tissues. It is best to remove the implant, and another operation is then required to remove the free silicone and/or to replace the implant.

Visible implants

The edge of the implant is sometimes obvious because of the lack of tissue between the implant and the thin remaining skin of the breast or even when the implant is placed behind the pectoralis major muscle (muscle on the front of the chest). This is a difficult problem to deal with. Various different methods are used, for example fat injections or the removal of the implant and reconstruction with a flap; however, none are entirely satisfactory.

Rippling/wrinkling

This is usually more obvious with saline-filled implants where the wrinkled shell of the implant and movement of the fluid is obvious beneath the skin. It is less common with silicone gel-filled implants that have a more viscous filler.

Local control – radiotherapy

Radiotherapy involves the use of ionizing radiation to destroy cancer cells. It can be delivered using beams generated by a linear accelerator (a machine that produces high energy X-rays (photons) or beams of electrons or, less commonly, gamma rays from a radioactive source).

Radiotherapy is directed to the specific areas that are most likely to contain cancer cells; the aim is to reduce the risk of the cancer recurring in that area (loco-regional recurrence, see page 124). Radiotherapy has become standard treatment after breast conserving surgery for all invasive breast cancers, high-grade non-invasive cancers and for some women after mastectomy. Adjuvant radiotherapy may also improve overall survival rates for breast cancer.

The specific areas that can be treated with radiotherapy are the:

- Remaining breast tissue (after breast conserving surgery)
- Chest wall (after mastectomy)
- Axilla
- Supraclavicular area (above the collar bone)
- Internal mammary chain (lymph glands beside the breast bone).

Remaining breast tissue

Adjuvant radiotherapy reduces the risk of local recurrence significantly when given after breast conserving surgery. The benefit depends on the size of tumour. For tumours smaller than 4 cm in diameter, the risk of local recurrence is reduced by as much as 75 per cent.

Chest wall

Even though nearly all breast tissue is removed after mastectomy, a significant number of women can develop loco-regional recurrence. The chest wall is the commonest area for a recurrence. It is likely that this is because cancer cells are left behind in the lymphatic channels in the skin and chest wall. Radiotherapy to the chest wall is of significant benefit in women with:

- A large primary tumour (larger than 5 cm)
- Four or more positive axillary lymph nodes
- A tumour involving the pectoralis major muscle or skin.

The role of radiotherapy in other cases is still being studied in clinical trials. For example, trials are looking at the benefit for women with high-grade tumours, where one to three axillary nodes are positive and where there is evidence of lymphovascular invasion.

Axilla

Radiotherapy to the axilla is of benefit for women with positive axillary nodes when a full axillary clearance (Levels 1–3) has not been performed. It is not recommended for women who have had a full axillary clearance because the risk of axillary recurrence is very low, and because the combination of axillary clearance and radiotherapy markedly increases the risk of lymphoedema (see page 74).

Supraclavicular area

For women who have four or more positive axillary lymph nodes, radiotherapy to the **supraclavicular** area is recommended. When fewer than four axillary nodes contain a tumour, there is no proven evidence to show that radiotherapy to the supraclavicular area is beneficial, although this is still being studied.

supraclavicular
Area above the collar bone.

Internal mammary chain

Clinical recurrence in these lymph nodes (situated behind the edge of the breast bone) is uncommon even when radiotherapy is not given. There is limited evidence to show whether radiotherapy is beneficial, and it remains a controversial area.

Radiotherapy methods

Radiotheropy can be given in different ways, as listed below.

External beam

Most breast cancer patients receive radiotherapy in this form. It is called 'external' because the device that delivers the radiotherapy is located some distance from the patient (see Colour Plate 16). The two common types of external beam radiation are photons and electrons. Photons are high-energy electromagnetic waves. Photons and electrons are generated through linear accelerators (machines that deliver radiotherapy). Electron therapy is used to 'boost' the radiation dose to the site of the primary tumour, whereas photons penetrate more deeply and are used to treat the whole breast.

Before therapy begins, patients have their treatment planned on a treatment simulator. The simulator looks similar to the treatment machine but, instead of delivering radiotherapy, takes X-ray pictures or a Computerized axial Tomography (CT) scan to visualize the area to be treated. This helps the radiotherapist to target the areas that need treatment and to minimize exposure to vital organs nearby like the lungs and heart. For the different areas that are treated, there are recognized regimes that deliver the dose of radiation in a number of individual sessions or 'fractions'. For treatment of the chest wall or entire breast, a typical total dose is 46–50 Gy. This is given in 23–25 fractions, where one fraction is given a day for five days of the week. The purpose of dividing up the total dose into smaller ones is to reduce the risk of tissue reactions (see below). There are different dose regimes with larger fractions given over a shorter period in order to reduce the number of visits to the hospital. Some patients will receive a 'boost', which is an additional dose to the tumour bed or to an area where the margins of excision are close.

Conventional external beam radiotherapy is usually given a few weeks after surgery, when the surgical wound has completely healed. If chemotherapy is also being recommended, radiotherapy usually follows this treatment. Typical regimes last three to five weeks (five days per week with a break at the weekend). Treatment lasts for a few minutes each day.

Q **I have had surgery and now need radiotherapy, chemotherapy and hormonal therapy. When and how will it all fit in together?**

A The usual sequence after surgery is to have chemotherapy followed by radiotherapy. Studies have shown that there is a better overall survival rate when chemotherapy is given before radiotherapy although the local recurrence rate may be higher. Hormonal therapy is usually started after completing chemotherapy.

Side effects of external beam radiotherapy

Side effects of external beam radiotherapy are few and usually temporary. They include skin reactions similar to sunburn (redness, dryness, sensitivity, sore, moist patches), and occasionally a cough and tiredness. The skin may become swollen and darker but this usually resolves after some months. Long-term damage to underlying organs and tissues such as the heart, lungs, bone, cartilage or nerves can happen years later but is very uncommon with modern treatment methods. Lymphoedema after surgery and radiotherapy occurs in less than 1 in 10 patients, although it is very rare for combined treatment to be recommended. The lymphoedema can be mild and hardly noticeable or may require treatment. In an extremely small number of cases, radiation-induced cancer can occur in the tissue that has been irradiated or in the nearby tissues at the margin of the radiotherapy field. However, the benefits from radiotherapy for the treatment of breast cancer far outweigh this rare risk.

Q **I have had a mastectomy. What is my risk of local recurrence with or without radiotherapy? Should I have radiotherapy?**

A The risk of local recurrence depends mostly on how many lymph nodes are involved and how big your tumour was. Other factors that influence it are margins of excision, grade of tumour, lymphovascular invasion, chest wall or skin involvement, and whether or not you will receive systemic adjuvant therapy (hormonal or chemotherapy). Ask your doctor what the likely benefits and risks are in your case and also to take into consideration any other illnesses you are suffering from.

Intraoperative radiotherapy

Intraoperative radiotherapy is a novel approach to treatment currently undergoing investigation. Radiotherapy is given while the patient is undergoing surgery for removal of the primary breast cancer. The machine that delivers the radiotherapy is brought into the operating theatre and the patient is treated while still under a general anaesthetic. High-dose radiotherapy is targeted at the remaining breast tissue before closure of the surgical wound. This method of delivery is not routinely offered and is not standard treatment in the UK or elsewhere in the world. It is currently undergoing clinical trials in the UK. Intraoperative radiotherapy is suitable for women who are having breast conserving surgery but not mastectomy. One advantage is that the X-rays do not have to pass through the skin and therefore the risk of skin damage is reduced. Another advantage is that it accurately targets the tumour bed, as the wound is still open. It also reduces the number of visits to the hospital after the surgery. Whether it is as effective as conventional external beam radiotherapy remains to be evaluated.

Brachytherapy

Brachytherapy (interstitial radiotherapy or plesiotherapy) involves the placement of radioactive implants inside the breast. The radioactive implants emit radiation that only affects the tissue close to the radioactive source. This method can be used to treat the tumour bed after surgery, the chest wall or, less commonly, it can be used as primary treatment for a breast cancer in a woman who will not have surgery. Radioactive implants are typically used in conjunction with external beam radiotherapy treatment.

At the time of surgery for removal of the lump (or at a later time), fine plastic tubes or a balloon catheter are placed into the breast tissue. The radioactive source is placed within these tubes or catheter and they are left in place for the duration of the treatment. The tubes or catheter are removed after the treatment has been completed. The rate of delivery of radioactivity to the tissue can be altered and treatment can be given in either a high dose or low dose. The radioactive source is placed into the tubes with remotely controlled automated devices to avoid handling by and exposure to medical personnel.

For low-dose delivery, treatment is on an in-patient basis in hospital, and the patient is isolated for the duration that the implants are in place because of the radioactivity. For high-dose delivery, treatment is on an out-patient basis.

Q I am likely to need radiotherapy after my mastectomy. Can I still have an immediate breast reconstruction?

A There are two issues concerning immediate breast reconstruction and radiotherapy. First, having an immediate reconstruction does not significantly affect the start date of radiotherapy. Second, the long-term cosmetic results of your breast reconstruction may be adversely affected by radiotherapy because there is an increased risk of capsular contracture if you have an implant reconstruction. You may be advised against having a free tissue flap transfer from your abdomen until after the radiotherapy in order to avoid irradiating the normal tissue of the flap which could affect the final cosmetic result.

Systemic therapy

Studies show that some women with early breast cancer who receive adjuvant systemic therapy in the form of hormonal therapy or chemotherapy have better outcomes in terms of longer survival and fewer recurrences. These drugs are also used for treatment of breast cancer that has returned or spread (see page 124).

When deciding on whether or not a woman with breast cancer should be given adjuvant systemic therapy, the following factors need to be considered:

- Risk of recurrence of breast cancer
- Potential benefits from the treatment
- Risks associated with the treatment
- The patient's willingness to put up with the effects of treatment balanced against the benefits.

Q My wound took a long time to heal and this delayed the start of my radiotherapy treatment for two months after the operation. Will this affect my outcome?

A Studies have shown that there is no significant difference to survival or local recurrence rates if there is a delay of up to eight weeks between surgery and adjuvant radiotherapy.

Hormonal (endocrine) treatment

Hormones (like oestrogen and progesterone) occur naturally in the body and act as chemical messengers. They control and promote the activity of normal cells in our bodies. A large proportion of breast cancers (70–80 per cent) contain within their cells an overabundance of the hormone receptors (HR) that bind to oestrogen and progesterone. These tumours are often dependent on oestrogen for their growth and reducing oestrogen can help prevent recurrence of the breast cancer. Breast cancer tissue is routinely tested for the presence of these receptors and, if found, are termed oestrogen receptor (ER) positive or progesterone receptor (PR) positive. Tumours may be positive for none, one or both receptors. Breast cancers in men are more frequently HR-positive compared to those in women.

The ovaries are the major source of oestrogen in pre-menopausal women. In post-menopausal women, however, the main source of oestrogen is from the conversion of male sex hormones (androgens) to oestrogen in tissues like fat, muscle, liver, adrenal and breast tissue. The conversion process involves a chemical enzyme called 'aromatase'. Drugs that block the action of aromatase are called 'aromatase inhibitors'. They lower the levels of oestrogen in post-menopausal women but have virtually no effect on lowering oestrogen levels in pre-menopausal women.

Hormonal treatment that either blocks the action of oestrogen or prevents the production of oestrogen is recommended for women who have HR-positive tumours. Such therapy is an effective form of treatment with relatively few side effects compared to chemotherapy.

In early stage breast cancers hormonal therapy reduces the risk of cancer recurrence as well as the incidence of a cancer arising in the opposite breast.

Hormonal manipulation is possible by:

- Ovarian suppression or ablation using surgery or radiation therapy (in premenopausal women)
- Drugs.

Ovarian ablation or suppression

The ovaries can be removed surgically or they can be made to stop functioning (producing oestrogen) by the use of drugs or radiotherapy.

Surgical removal of ovaries (oophorectomy) provides a permanent and rapid onset of oestrogen withdrawal. Modern laparoscopic oophorectomy (the use of keyhole surgery to remove the ovaries) is simpler and faster than conventional methods and has fewer complications. Surgical removal of the ovaries reduces the incidence of ovarian cancer in women who have a high risk of both breast and ovarian cancer (for example altered BRCA1 gene carriers). As a single treatment, **ovarian ablation** provides a significant reduction in the risk of recurrence, and a significant improvement in survival for pre-menopausal women with breast cancer.

ovarian ablation or suppression
Stopping the ovaries from producing oestrogen.

Ovarian ablation using radiation therapy is safe with few side effects. Oestrogen levels are reduced more slowly as compared with surgical removal. It can be done on an out-patient basis but this method has now largely been surpassed by the use of drugs.

LHRH (Luteinizing Hormone Releasing Hormone) agonists

LHRH agonist
A drug that mimics Luteinizing Hormone Releasing Hormone (LHRH) that acts by reducing the amount of circulating oestrogen in the body.

Goserelin (Zoladex®)

Goserelin acts by reducing the stimulus that makes the ovaries produce oestrogen. It is used for the management of advanced breast cancer and also, occasionally, as an alternative or supplement to chemotherapy for ER-positive early breast cancer in pre-menopausal women. It has a reversible action and may preserve a woman's fertility (but this is still under study). As it is reversible, the side effects of long-term oestrogen deficiency are reduced. The optimal duration of therapy is not yet known but for early breast cancer it is often given for two years. Goserelin is given as a sub-cutaneous injection (just under the skin) every four weeks.

Part of the beneficial effect of chemotherapy is thought to be due to the suppressive effect that it has on the ovaries. Trials have shown that the combination of ovarian suppression or ablation and tamoxifen is equivalent to an older form of chemotherapy for pre-menopausal women with ER-positive tumours. Whether this approach is as effective as more modern chemotherapy is not yet known. Trials are underway to find out the value of ovarian suppression or ablation for young women who, having received chemotherapy, did not become post-menopausal afterwards.

Drugs that suppress hormones

Apart from the methods available to stop the ovaries from producing oestrogen, drugs are available that suppress the hormonal effects of oestrogen, by blocking the uptake of oestrogen by cancer cells or reducing the production of oestrogen in other tissues. They are used for women with ER- or PR-positive tumours. Examples of drugs used in hormonal therapy include:

- Anti oestrogens – tamoxifen (Nolvadex®), toremifene, fulvestrant (Faslodex®)
- Aromatase inhibitors – anastrazole (Arimidex®), letrozole (Femara®), exemestane (Aromasin®), formestane

- Progestogens – megesterol acetate, medroxyprogesterone. (Progestogens are not commonly used anymore because the more modern drugs have fewer side effects and are more effective.)

Q Why are some of the drugs known by different names?

A European Law requires the use of the Recommended International Non-proprietary Name for medicines. This is the generic name of the drug. When a drug company discovers a drug and manufactures it, it gives it a proprietary name to identify it as coming from that particular company. For example tamoxifen (generic name) is also known as Soltamox® and Nolvadex-D® (proprietary name).

Adjuvant hormonal therapy after surgery for primary breast cancer is usually recommended for five years. Sometimes cancer cells build up resistance to a certain drug and it becomes ineffective. Other hormonal drugs may still be effective. It may be beneficial to change to a different drug after a period of two to three years. Studies are currently underway that look at switching to another hormone drug such as anastrazole or exemestane after using tamoxifen. Women should ask their oncologist if there is a trial that they might be suitable to take part in, or if there is any new evidence to show that they might benefit from changing their drug therapy.

For early stage breast cancer the drugs most commonly used are tamoxifen (pre- and post-menopausal women) or one of the aromatase inhibitors (post-menopausal women). Of the aromatase inhibitors, exemestane can be used after two to three years of tamoxifen. Anastrazole is licensed as an alternative to tamoxifen for post-menopausal women with early breast cancer and for women who have a contraindication to tamoxifen, for example if they have a high risk of blood clots or abnormalities in the endometrium (womb). Letrozole can be used for women who have already received standard adjuvant tamoxifen. More evidence is emerging all the time about the benefits of these and other new drugs, which may enable more women to use them.

Anti oestrogens

Tamoxifen

This is a man-made drug and has been widely and successfully used for the treatment of women of all ages and with any cancer stage who have HR-positive breast cancers. There is no benefit for women with HR-negative tumours. Standard treatment for early breast cancer is 20 mg per day for five years. It has been found to significantly reduce the risk of local recurrence, to prolong survival and to reduce the rate of a cancer appearing in the other breast. There are other benefits to taking tamoxifen including a possible reduced risk of heart disease and preservation of bone strength (for post-menopausal women).

Side effects of tamoxifen include:

- Hot flushes
- Vaginal discharge or irritation
- Ovarian cysts (benign)
- An increased risk of thrombosis in the deep veins of the leg (Deep Venous Thrombosis – DVT) and pulmonary emboli (clots in the lungs) in less than 1 in 100 women
- An increased risk of endometrial cancer (cancer of the womb); there are one or two deaths per 1000 women from endometrial cancer after ten years of taking tamoxifen – women taking tamoxifen should have tests if they have unusual bleeding from the womb or new vaginal discharge

- Rarely eye problems such as cataracts (rare) and retinopathy (damage to the back of the eye affecting eyesight).

While taking tamoxifen, women are advised not to become pregnant as tamoxifen could potentially harm the developing baby.

Q I have heard on the news that there is a new drug called Arimidex® (anastrazole) that is more effective than tamoxifen. Why hasn't my doctor given me that instead of tamoxifen?

A Anastrazole is an aromatase inhibitor and only suitable for post-menopausal women with tumours that are ER-positive. Early results from ATAC (Arimidex or Tamoxifen Alone or in Combination) trial have shown there is an additional benefit in reducing relapse rates for women taking anastrazole instead of tamoxifen, but the follow-up period has only been five years. Longer term results are awaited to see if there is a real benefit to survival rates. Keep asking your oncologist or surgeon about the latest evidence from clinical trials as it emerges and ask whether you should change your hormonal therapy.

Aromatase inhibitors

Aromatase inhibitors are man-made drugs that interfere with the production or action of oestrogen in the body by inhibiting the enzyme aromatase. They slow or stop the growth of breast cancer in post-menopausal women with ER-positive tumours. They are not useful in pre-menopausal women in whom the main source of oestrogen is from their ovaries. Examples of aromatase inhibitors are as follows.

Anastrazole

Anastrazole can be considered for post-menopausal women with early stage breast cancer, those who have a contraindication to taking tamoxifen, or who have a recurrence of breast cancer while taking tamoxifen, or after finishing a course of tamoxifen. Anastrazole is taken as a tablet once a day.

Q I have been treated for breast cancer. Can I use local oestrogens for vaginal dryness?

A We do not know for sure what the risks are of using local oestrogens for a woman with breast cancer. Local oestrogens can be applied in the form of a vaginal tablet, vaginal ring or vaginal cream, and all of them can help with vaginal dryness. The smallest effective dose should be used in order to minimize the risks from the oestrogen being absorbed into the bloodstream. In short, you should weigh up the risk of getting a relapse or a new cancer against your symptoms, and how it affects your quality of life after a careful discussion with your oncologist.

Letrozole

Letrozole is sometimes used as preoperative treatment for post-menopausal women with localized breast cancer in order to shrink the tumour prior to surgery. It can also be used for women who have received prior standard adjuvant tamoxifen for early breast cancer, and for advanced cancer where tamoxifen or another hormonal drug has failed.

Other aromatase inhibitors are currently in use for women with advanced breast cancer and are being studied in clinical trials for women with primary breast cancer (see page 131).

There are many drugs that are currently being developed and undergoing clinical trials for the treatment of breast cancer. Ask your oncologist about the latest developments and any clinical trials that you may benefit from taking part in.

Q Can I use Hormone Replacement Therapy (HRT) at all with a diagnosis of breast cancer?

A HRT is contraindicated (not advised) in women with breast cancer.

Women with a diagnosis of breast cancer have a higher risk of a cancer arising in their opposite breast and for those who have residual breast tissue after breast conserving surgery, there is a risk of local recurrence in their treated breast. While it seems illogical to increase the risk of a relapse of breast cancer by taking something that is known to put women at risk, it becomes a quality of life issue as to whether or not you can put up with your menopausal symptoms. There are clinical trials underway that are looking at whether or not there is an accelerated rate of relapse or death in women who have a history of breast cancer and who are exposed to HRT.

Q What is tibolone?

A Tibolone (Livial™) is a synthetic steroid with oestrogenic effects used for menopausal symptoms (hot flushes, night sweats, vaginal soreness and dryness). It does increase the risk of breast cancer but to a lesser extent than combined oestrogen and progesterone HRT preparations.

Q I do not have breast cancer but wonder if I should be taking HRT if it increases the risk of getting breast cancer?

A In women who have not had breast cancer, HRT is appropriate for the symptoms of menopause that include hot flushes, night sweats and vaginal soreness and dryness. HRT also helps lessen post-menopausal osteoporosis but other drugs are preferred. HRT does not reduce the incidence of coronary heart disease and should not be taken for this purpose. HRT does increase the risk of deep venous thrombosis, pulmonary embolism, stroke, endometrial cancer and breast cancer. There are data to show that there is a small but significant risk of breast cancer in women (without a diagnosis of breast cancer) who take HRT for more than 5 years. The risk becomes higher the longer a woman takes it. Combined oestrogen/progesterone HRT preparations have a higher risk than those that contain oestrogen alone. You should discuss the pros and cons of HRT with your doctor in order to make a decision about taking it.

Chemotherapy

cytotoxic drug
Drug that kills an actively dividing cell.

Chemotherapy is a form of systemic (whole body) therapy that uses **cytotoxic drugs** to kill cancer cells. These drugs act on all actively dividing cells in the body and are particularly effective on cancer cells because they divide very quickly. The various groups of cytotoxic drugs work by killing cells in different ways. When two or more of these drugs are combined as part of a chemotherapy regime, they often work more effectively than a single drug, giving a better response, lower rate of drug resistance and better survival. The major drawback of using cytotoxic drugs is that they damage both normal and cancer cells. When they are used at the correct dose levels and intervals, normal cells will recover. It is the need for this 'window' for recovery of normal cells that determines the schedule for giving the drug. Chemotherapy drugs are normally given at three to four week intervals and each interval is called a 'cycle'.

intravenously
Injection into a vein.

Chemotherapy drugs are usually given **intravenously** through a cannula (small thin plastic tube) inserted into a vein in the arm (see Colour Plate 17). The tube is usually taken out after the drugs are administered and a new one put in for the next cycle. Sometimes it is more practical to insert a longer thin plastic tube into a larger vein in the neck or just beneath the collarbone and have the other end come out through the skin of the chest wall (Hickmann line or Groshong line). A Peripherally Inserted Central Catheter (PICC) line is a long thin catheter that is inserted through the vein at the bend in the elbow and the other end lies in one of the large veins going towards the heart. A PortaCath is based on the same principle but has an injection port that is situated beneath the skin on the chest wall so that the tube is not visible on the skin surface.

For breast cancer, chemotherapy is used in three main situations:

- Adjuvant therapy after surgery or radiotherapy
- Primary or **neoadjuvant therapy** (before surgery)
- Advanced or metastatic breast cancer.

neoadjuvant therapy
Additional therapy that is given before surgery.

Q What benefit will I get from chemotherapy? And how does my oncologist decide which drugs are best for me?

A This is an important question to ask your oncologist because the benefit is different for each individual woman. It is your age, menopausal status, the function of your heart, kidneys, liver and general health that will be considered as well as the size, grade, hormone receptor (HR) status of your tumour, presence or not of lymphovascular invasion, and any evidence of spread in the nodes or spread of the cancer around your body. Your oncologist will decide on a drug or regime that suits your individual case.

Adjuvant chemotherapy

Adjuvant chemotherapy is used after surgery for early breast cancer in order to destroy any clinically undetectable cancer cells that may have spread outside the breast through the bloodstream or lymphatics. It is given as an insurance policy so that the chance of relapse in another part of the body is reduced. It is usually given before radiotherapy but can be given afterwards. Women who gain most benefit from adjuvant chemotherapy include those where:

- The lymph nodes are involved
- The tumour is larger than 2 cm in diameter
- The tumour is grade 3 (it looks aggressive under the microscope)

- The woman is young (younger than 35 years)
- There is lymphovascular invasion (tumour cells found in the lymphatic and blood vessels in the breast)
- The tumour cells do not express the oestrogen receptor (ER-negative tumours that do not respond to hormonal therapy).

Lymph node involvement is the most important risk factor for relapse of breast cancer. It shows that cancer cells have spread outside the breast through the lymphatic system and there is a risk of some cancer cells also having left the breast through the blood vessels.

Q I want to know what my chances are with and without chemotherapy. Where can I get this information?

A Your oncologist is the best person to discuss this with you. He or she will take into account your age, size and grade of your tumour, the number of lymph nodes involved if any, and whether or not your tumour is hormone receptor- HR-positive. You may also obtain information from the internet from www.mayoclinic.com and log on to the section on 'Treatment Decisions' and Adjuvant therapy for breast cancer' and 'Your own chances'. You can use the calculator that will give estimated figures of your own chances of surviving the next ten years without the cancer coming back. Remember that these figures are only an estimate and your prognosis may be different from the figures given in the tool. It is very important that you discuss your individual treatment plan with your oncologist.

The degree of benefit that a woman will gain from chemotherapy depends on her individual case. Women who are pre-menopausal and who have involved lymph nodes gain the most benefit from chemotherapy. The benefits are even greater for women whose tumours have the highest risk of relapse. Part of the beneficial effect from chemotherapy is thought to be because it brings on the menopause and stops the ovaries from producing female hormones (see page 104)

Women over the age of 50 also benefit, but probably to a lesser extent. Again, the benefit to an individual woman will depend on the characteristics of her particular cancer. Some women with HR positive disease may only have a small benefit. It is a value judgement for each individual woman whether the benefit outweighs the side effects of the therapy or not. The decision is often quite complex and will require a discussion with the oncologist to determine the risk:benefit ratio in each case.

Chemotherapy drug regimes

Some of the more common drug combinations for treating breast cancer in the UK are listed below. This list is not comprehensive and women may be offered a different drug regime or one that is being studied as part of a clinical trial. The most common chemotherapy regime used for adjuvant therapy and for the treatment of advanced disease used to be CMF (Cyclophosphamide, Methotrexate, 5-Fluorouracil). However, this combination has largely been replaced by regimes containing a class of drugs known as the **anthracyclines**. Combinations containing an anthracycline drug generally show better results than have been obtained with CMF.

The various drugs cause different side effects and have different toxic effects. The decision about a certain regime depends on the individual patient,

anthracyclines
A group of cytotoxic antibiotic drugs that include doxorubicin and epirubicin among others. Mitoxantrone (mitozantrone) is a derivative of this group.

taking into account the risks of the treatment, any pre-existing illnesses and the balance between the risks of taking the drug and the likely benefit.

Q What dose of drugs will I be given?

A Data from clinical trials looking at different drug doses show that for most cytotoxic drugs there is a dose at which there is maximal benefit, but a higher dose will not give a better result and can cause more toxic effects. Should you experience an infection associated with a low white blood cell count, severe nausea or vomiting or severe mouth ulcers, your chemotherapy may be delayed or the dose may be altered.

Chemotherapy combinations used for adjuvant treatment are:

- FEC (Flourouracil, Epirubicin, Cyclophosphamide)
- AC (Adriamycin® [Doxorubicin], Cyclophosphamide)
- CMF (Cyclophosphamide, Methotrexate, 5-Fluorouracil).

Primary (neoadjuvant) chemotherapy

Primary or neoadjuvant chemotherapy is given before surgery or radiotherapy. There is no difference in recurrence or survival rates when comparing adjuvant versus neoadjuvant chemotherapy. Primary chemotherapy can be offered in these situations:

- Large tumour where it is felt that mastectomy would be necessary
- Inflammatory cancer
- Locally advanced breast cancer.

Advantages of having neoadjuvant chemotherapy are:

- There is a higher chance of preserving the breast in some women whose tumours shrink to a small enough size to allow breast conserving surgery as opposed to mastectomy
- A locally advanced cancer may become operable
- The way in which the tumour responds to chemotherapy gives a prediction of survival outcome in the long term
- Different chemotherapy drugs can be used if the tumour does not respond to a particular regime.

Advanced breast cancer and chemotherapy

Chemotherapy for patients with metastatic or locally advanced cancer is aimed at relief of symptoms, improving quality of life, and prolonging life where possible. When a breast cancer is locally advanced and inoperable, chemotherapy can be effective in shrinking the tumour. There are many different cytotoxic drugs licensed for advanced breast cancer. They can be given in different combinations and in different treatment regimes. Combinations are usually only a little more effective than single drugs given on their own, but they can have more side effects.

Q What is a 'very high dose chemotherapy regime'?

A The concept of using very high doses was based on experimental laboratory findings that showed that in the test tube very high doses of certain drugs (five to ten times the normal dose) could overcome resistance of breast cancer cells. At present there

 is no evidence to show that there is a real benefit to women with this type of regime. Because the doses of the drugs are so high, the treatment causes death of the bone marrow cells that normally produce blood cells. Special bone marrow or stem cell support is necessary for these women and they are at risk of severe infection. This approach has not shown any advantages over the normal doses of chemotherapy.

Side effects of chemotherapy

Cytotoxic drugs do not only act specifically on cancer cells, and therefore some of the normal cells in the bone marrow, hair follicles and lining of the gut and bladder can be affected as well. This is why chemotherapy can sometimes cause unpleasant side effects. Many people, however, only experience a few and they can usually be well controlled with medication. Some of the commoner short-term side effects are detailed below.

Bone marrow suppression

It is important for women to realize that nearly all chemotherapy drugs can cause bone marrow suppression. This commonly happens seven to ten days after administration of chemotherapy. Because white cells (help fight infection), platelets (for blood clotting) and red cells (transport oxygen around the body) are manufactured in the bone marrow there is a reduced number of these cells in the circulation, thereby causing:

- Lowered resistance to infection – regular blood counts are taken before each cycle of chemotherapy, and if the white cell count is very low and an infection suspected, antibiotics will be given. The chemotherapy cycle may be delayed until the blood cell counts rise again. Granulocyte Colony Stimulating Factor (GCSF) is a drug that can be given to stimulate the bone marrow to produce white cells. It reduces the length of time the bone marrow usually takes to recover. It is extremely important that if there are symptoms of feeling hot or unwell, any flu-like symptoms or signs of a fever (38°c or above), that the hospital is contacted immediately because these are signs of an infection. This is most likely to happen around day seven to ten of the chemotherapy cycle. Intravenous antibiotics (administered through a vein) must be started immediately if there is any suspicion of an infection.

- Low platelet count – signs of a low platelet count are nosebleeds, bruising, unexplained bleeding and constant headaches. The commonest time for the blood counts to drop is in the middle of a chemotherapy cycle. It occurs very rarely with standard doses of chemotherapy.
- Anaemia – tiredness, lethargy, dizziness and breathlessness are signs of anaemia. Treatment is by blood transfusion or, much less commonly, epoitin (recombinant human erythropoetin)– a drug that stimulates the production of red cells and shortens the period of anaemia.

Nausea and vomiting

These can be distressing and are best prevented. There are effective medications for nausea and vomiting. The medications are usually given before the start of chemotherapy and for a few days afterwards. They should be taken regularly for best effect. If one drug does not work, women should ask for a different type as others are available. Eating small frequent meals may help reduce vomiting. Eating foods from the fridge can reduce any nausea brought on by strong food smells.

Sore mouth and mouth ulcers

This is a common complication of chemotherapy and is more likely to happen with anthracyclines, flourouracil and methotrexate. Using a soft toothbrush and fluoride toothpaste after meals and before bed is essential in order to try to prevent mouth ulcers. Mouthwashes after meals and before bed may be necessary if there are ulcers in the mouth. To protect or soothe a sore area, there are products such as orabase or sucralfate that can give relief. For pain, gel applied directly to the ulcer or liquid analgesic gargles are helpful. Nutritious drinks, soups or liquidized food are easier to take than solids. Pineapple stimulates the production of saliva and can be helpful. Citrus fruits or juices and spicy foods should be avoided. It is advisable to avoid having any major dental work done while undergoing chemotherapy.

Hair loss

Hair loss is more common with certain chemotherapy drugs. These include epirubicin, docetaxel, paclitaxel and doxorubicin. Sometimes hair loss can be prevented or lessened by using a method called scalp cooling. A very cold cap is worn over the head when the chemotherapy drugs are being given. Some women suffer with headaches when they use the cold cap. Hair loss normally starts about two to four weeks after the first cycle, and the hair may thin or it may be lost completely. The eyelashes, eyebrows and other body hair may also be lost. A breast care nurse can arrange for women to obtain a wig before chemotherapy starts. The hair will grow again after the end of chemotherapy but may be of a different colour and texture. Patients are advised not to use strong chemicals such as hair dyes or perms for at least six months after the completion of chemotherapy because the hair can be damaged and the uptake of chemicals is not predictable.

Premature menopause

The risk of premature menopause rises in older women, with longer courses of chemotherapy, and is more common with cyclophosphamide. Up to 40 per cent of women having chemotherapy have an early menopause. The periods can stop temporarily and some women have their periods return as long as 18 months after the end of chemotherapy.

Reproductive function

Most cytotoxic drugs will damage a foetus, and the risk is highest in the first trimester of pregnancy. Contraceptive advice should be sought and contraception used even if a woman's periods stop during treatment. Barrier methods of contraception (condoms or diaphragm with a spermicide) are the most suitable during the course of chemotherapy. A premature menopause may affect fertility in a woman. If a woman remains fertile after chemotherapy, there is no known increase in risk of abortion or of foetal abnormalities in future pregnancies.

Q I have breast cancer, am pregnant and will need chemotherapy. What will happen to my baby?

A Your doctors will discuss the effect of chemotherapy on your baby and on your overall predicted outcome. You may be advised to terminate the pregnancy and this will depend on the stage of your pregnancy, the risk of toxic effects from chemotherapy to your unborn baby, and how much benefit you will expect to gain from having it. If you are in your second or third trimester of pregnancy, you should discuss with your obstetrician and oncologist the risks and benefits of early delivery of your baby versus continuing with the pregnancy and the effect of chemotherapy on your baby. Your prognosis will not be altered by termination of pregnancy. Your periods may stop and you may have an early menopause after chemotherapy especially if you are older than 30.

Fatigue

All chemotherapy drugs can cause fatigue. It is more common as treatment progresses, and may last for several months after the end of the course of chemotherapy. Patients often feel better when they do gentle exercise regularly. It is useful to achieve a balance between the amount of activity and rest on a daily basis.

Diarrhoea

This happens to some women and usually settles with anti-diarrhoeal medications.

Constipation

This is more commonly due to the drugs given to prevent sickness and vomiting rather than the chemotherapy drugs themselves. A high fluid intake, high fibre diet and gentle exercise is recommended. Gentle laxatives can be prescribed if necessary.

Thrombosis and pulmonary embolism

Although the risk of thrombosis in the deep veins of the leg or pelvis is increased by having both cancer and chemotherapy, it is uncommon. Signs of a leg thrombosis are swelling and pain in the leg(s). If a part of the clot in the deep veins breaks off into the bloodstream, it usually lodges in the lung and can cause a pulmonary embolism. This is a serious condition. A symptom of pulmonary embolism is breathlessness. Patients should contact their doctors if they have any of these complaints.

Damage to the veins

Some darkening of the veins in the arm is normal and is of no consequence in itself as the colour will fade after the completion of chemotherapy. Sometimes the veins become sore or hardened because of the damage to the lining, and clots form within them. The veins may resemble a cord; they do not usually cause any harm and settle down after several months. Should any of the cytotoxic drugs extravasate (leak) into the tissue surrounding the vein where they are administered, damage and irritation of that tissue may occur. It is important for women to immediately report any pain and stinging, swelling or leakage around the infusion site while their chemotherapy is being administered, so that prompt action can be taken in order to prevent the spread of the drug into the surrounding tissue.

Chemotherapy nurses are highly experienced in drug administration and will regularly assess the injection site for any signs of leakage. When it is difficult to locate a suitable vein in an arm, the use of a longer thin plastic tube into a larger vein in the neck or just beneath the collarbone may become necessary (see page 110).

Damage to the heart

Doxorubicin (Adriamycin®) has been reported to cause damage to the heart. The risks of heart damage are small when the recommended dose is not exceeded. An ECG (electrocardiogram or tracing of the electrical activity of the heart) is routinely done for all patients receiving an anthracycline drug. A cardiac (heart) function test is recommended for older women and those with a history of heart disease. The combination of trastuzumab with anthracyclines has been found to have a higher incidence of damage to the heart and so this combination is no longer used.

Cystitis

Cyclophosphamide can rarely cause a complication called haemorrhagic cystitis (cystitis associated with blood in the urine). Women are advised to drink 2–3 litres of fluid per day to avoid it. Any sensation of burning or stinging on passing urine must be reported.

Discoloration of the urine

As the anthracycline group of drugs is coloured red, the urine may also become red when women first pass urine after the infusion, and this is not a result of any bleeding.

Other cancers

Other cancers like leukaemias are rarely caused by chemotherapy. The incidence is less than 1 in 100 patients. The benefit of chemotherapy for the treatment of breast cancer far outweighs this small risk.

Q I need to have chemotherapy and hormonal therapy for treatment of my breast cancer. I am concerned that my periods may not come back afterwards and that I will be infertile. What are my options for having a baby in the future?

A The risk of you becoming infertile will depend on your age and the type of systemic therapy you receive. If the risk of infertility is high, there may be several options open to you and the success rates are variable. Some of these options include harvesting a few of your own eggs, in vitro fertilization (if you have a partner) and frozen storage of the fertilized eggs, or harvesting some of your ovarian tissue for frozen storage (if you do not have a partner). Both of these methods are intended for future use. A disadvantage of the method of using frozen storage of fertilized eggs is that the process takes time and there will be a delay to the start of chemotherapy. Another potential disadvantage is that egg collection involves stimulating the ovaries and the effect of ovarian stimulation may potentially stimulate the cancer to grow. The use of frozen ovarian tissue is still experimental despite a report in the Lancet (a medical journal) in 2004 of a child being born using this method. Discuss the pros and cons of the options available to you with your oncologist.

Follow-up after treatment for breast cancer

As there is a chance that breast cancer may recur, women have follow-up appointments with breast cancer specialists (surgeon, oncologist, specialist nurse) at regular intervals. The chance of recurrence is highest in the first two years after treatment, and most follow-up protocols are designed towards this. For example, women are encouraged to do monthly breast self-examinations (and to report any changes to their doctors), have a clinical examination every three to six months for three years, then every six to twelve months for two years, then annually. In addition, a two yearly mammogram is recommended and in future, follow-up may be handed over to the general practitioner for women who remain well three years after their initial treatment. There is no evidence to show that any other investigations or tests, such as blood tests or scans, are of any benefit unless there is a specific problem. Patients have open access to their breast care nurse who is available for support and advice. The nurses can arrange appropriate appointments for women who experience new symptoms or who have any concerns in between their routine appointments.

Recurrent breast cancer

Long-term follow-up studies of women who have been treated for breast cancer show that women may survive even if their breast cancer recurs. The likelihood of recurrence depends on various factors related to the original tumour and what treatment was given. Most recurrences happen in the first two to three years after initially being diagnosed. Relapse of breast cancer can happen either locally in the area of the original tumour, as metastases or as a combination of both. When a breast cancer recurs, it is usually in the region of the original tumour and is known as a local recurrence. The aim of treatment depends on whether or not there is evidence of systemic spread in the form of metastases.

For locally recurrent cancers and where there is no evidence of metastases, treatment is aimed at local control. The same therapies apply as for primary treatment and include surgery or radiotherapy. The choice of what can be offered depends on whether the recurrence is small and can be removed surgically or whether it is more advanced. Radiotherapy cannot usually be given a second time if it was given as part of primary treatment because of the risk of damage to normal tissues. If the recurrent tumour can be removed by surgery, this can be done again. For some women, following removal of the tumour and surrounding tissue, a reconstructive procedure may be necessary in the form of a skin graft or flap of tissue in order to fill in and cover the defect.

Systemic therapy is often started (if not previously given) when a recurrence occurs or is changed if a women was already on such therapy. This takes the form of hormonal therapy or chemotherapy, depending on the age of the patient, HR status of the tumour, pre-existing illnesses and individual patient preferences and factors.

Recurrent DCIS is treated with further surgery. Breast conserving surgery may be possible if radiotherapy has not previously been given. Radiotherapy cannot be given a second time because it would cause damage to normal tissues. Mastectomy is usually necessary if previous treatment was with radiotherapy, and for widespread disease.

When a breast cancer recurs in the form of metastases, it is known as 'advanced' breast cancer. Recurrence in the form of metastases can be treated. Treatment is aimed at relieving symptoms, improving quality of life, and prolonging life where possible. If the recurrence has occurred while the woman is still receiving adjuvant systemic therapy, this therapy is altered to a different drug(s). Breast cancer is best considered as a manageable chronic illness. Many drugs are available for treatment and new ones are emerging all the time. Modern methods of radiotherapy produce fewer side effects. Modern anaesthesia has made surgery safer and it can therefore be offered to more women.

Q I have a recurrence of the cancer in my breast. It is a small lump just under the scar. I previously had a wide local excision followed by radiotherapy. What are my treatment options?

A A local recurrence on its own can be treated with surgery to remove the recurrent cancer. This is usually in the form of a mastectomy because you cannot have radiotherapy to the same area a second time and radiotherapy is usually needed to treat the remaining breast tissue. You will be checked to see if you have any evidence of metastases that can be treated with hormonal therapy (if your tumour is HR positive) or with chemotherapy.

Advanced breast cancer

The term 'advanced breast cancer' is broad and includes women with:

- Locally advanced disease
- Metastatic spread.

Advanced breast cancers are those that have spread into the overlying skin, underlying muscle, axillary or internal mammary lymph nodes or have spread into the bloodstream to distant sites to form metastases. Treatment is tailored to each individual patient for local or systemic control and can include surgery, radiotherapy, chemotherapy, hormonal therapy or other newer drugs alone or in combination.

When a breast cancer first shows at an advanced stage (Stage III or IV, see Chapter 2, pages 30–31), the chance of cure is unlikely, and treatment is aimed at relieving symptoms, improving quality of life, and prolonging life where possible.

While most women with metastatic breast cancer will eventually die of their disease, some women do live for several years. It has been shown that over 70 per cent of women with a diagnosis of metastatic breast cancer are not limited in their normal daily routine and are effectively living with their diagnosis. Many patients are able to manage their illness as a chronic disease and maintain an active and satisfying work, family and personal life for several years.

my experience

I have metastatic breast cancer in my spine, my lungs and my liver. It recurred when I was 19 weeks' pregnant with my second child. I started chemotherapy in my twentieth week of pregnancy. They induced me at 36 weeks and I now have a delightful one-year old who has more energy than I can cope with. I have a child minder who comes in for four hours a day so that I can have a lie down in the afternoons after picking up my four-year old from school. I started on epirubicin while still pregnant (it doesn't harm the baby in the womb), docetaxel after the birth, and am now on Herceptin and Capecitabine. My tummy is so bloated with fluid that people think I am at least seven months pregnant again. We live in a shared house at the moment and I am looking forward to us getting our own home, as it is very cramped with the two children. My dream is for us to sit around our own kitchen table to have breakfast together, just the four of us.

Local treatment for advanced breast cancer

Surgery

Surgery can be helpful to remove painful or ulcerating breast lesions. Total mastectomy involves removal of the whole breast and the cancer, with the intention of reducing the tumour load, but not necessarily all of the tumour cells. It aims to reduce pain or discomfort and to make the area easier to manage. A reconstructive procedure may be necessary in the form of a flap of tissue or skin graft to close the defect left from removal of the tumour.

Q What is a Stage III breast cancer?

A The TNM (Tumour, Node, Metastases) staging system for breast cancer has four stages. A Stage III breast cancer is one that is large (larger than 5 cm) or with large or positive lymph nodes or where the tumour is stuck to the underlying muscle or has ulcerated through the skin.

Q What is a Stage IV breast cancer?

A According to the TNM (Tumour, Node, Metastases) staging system, Stage IV breast cancer is one that has metastasized outside the breast. It can be of any size, and the lymph glands often contain tumour.

Radiotherapy

Radiotherapy to a locally advanced breast tumour may be possible and preferable to surgery if the risk of surgery outweighs the benefits in someone who has another illness as well as the breast cancer. Radiotherapy can also be combined with surgery and given after a total mastectomy.

Systemic treatment for advanced breast cancer

When the breast cancer has spread to other parts of the body, endocrine drugs, chemotherapy or other drugs (trastuzumab and bisphosphonates) can be used to shrink the metastases and improve symptoms.

Chemotherapy

Combination chemotherapy can be useful in controlling the advanced cancer locally and improving symptoms from metastases. If chemotherapy was not given as adjuvant therapy originally, the first-line combinations of cytotoxic drugs are used (see page 113). If chemotherapy was given as part of the treatment of the original cancer there are still many other drugs that can be offered. A second-line drug regime would include a different drug, for example, docetaxel (a taxane).

Some chemotherapy drugs are effective when given on their own. They can be given if they have not previously been used as part of a regime and include the following:

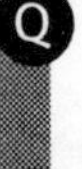

What is first-line treatment? What is second-line treatment?

A First-line drugs are those that are used in the first instance for treatment. They are known to be the most effective ones with the fewest toxic effects. Second- and third-line drugs are used when breast cancer recurs and are not as effective and may have more severe side effects.

Capecitabine

Capecitabine is broken down in the body to fluorouracil and is used for locally advanced or metastatic breast cancer. It is sometimes combined with docetaxel where anthracyclines are unsuitable or have not worked. It can also be used alone when anthracyclines and taxanes have failed or cannot be given again. This drug is taken in tablet form at home. The palms of the hands and soles of the feet may become red and sore (hand-foot syndrome). A glycerine-based hand cream is useful for this. Some women experience a metallic taste in their mouth while on this drug. Diarrhoea and vomiting are common side effects.

Taxanes

Docetaxel (Taxotere®) and paclitaxel (Taxol®) are in this group of drugs. Taxanes are used where initial chemotherapy regimes have failed or where they are not appropriate. Docetaxel and paclitaxel can cause an allergic reaction and tend to result in nausea and vomiting, and they are therefore given with dexamethasone (a steroid) in order to reduce the risk. These drugs cause mouth ulcers and hair loss, usually three to four weeks after the first dose. Women are advised to obtain a wig before the start of their chemotherapy if they wish to use one. Some women experience numbness or pins and needles in their fingers or toes that usually resolves after the completion of chemotherapy. Docetaxel can cause discoloration of the fingernails and, very occasionally, women may lose their nails. Diarrhoea is sometimes a side effect and can be treated with medication.

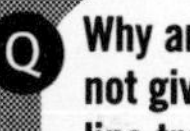

Q Why are taxanes not given as first-line treatment?

A Taxanes cause more short-term side effects than first-line drugs. To date, the added benefit with the use of a taxane drug appears to be small compared to conventional regimes.

Epirubicin (Pharmorubicin®)

As epirubicin is coloured red, the urine may become red also. In addition to the general side effects of all chemotherapy drugs, epirubicin can also cause diarrhoea and it is necessary for women to keep themselves well hydrated by drinking lots of fluids. Medicines can be taken to control the diarrhoea. Epirubicin can interfere with liver function. Blood tests are taken before the start of chemotherapy and before each cycle to ensure that the liver can cope with this drug.

Vinorelbine (Navelbine®)

Vinorelbine can cause reversible damage to nerves that results in numbness of the fingers and motor weakness. Recovery is usually slow but complete. Vinorelbine also causes hair loss, abdominal pain and constipation or diarrhoea.

Other drugs include the following:

Immunotherapy

Monoclonal antibody therapy

Trastuzumab (Herceptin®) is an antibody drug that works by blocking the stimulus to breast cancer cells that are overly sensitive to a particular naturally occurring growth factor called HER2. About 15–25 per cent of women have this type of breast cancer. Trastuzumab is a second-line chemotherapy drug. It has shown promising results when combined with anthracyline and taxane-based chemotherapy drugs for metastatic breast cancer. Clinical trials are underway that are looking at trastuzumab for early breast cancer. Side effects include chills, fever, allergic reactions, damage to the heart, muscle and joint pain and low blood pressure. The heart should be monitored before and during treatment.

Bisphosphonates

These drugs reduce the rate of bone turnover and help in the prevention and treatment of high calcium levels in the blood (hypercalcaemia) caused by bony metastases. Examples in this group include zoledronic acid (Zometa®), sodium clodronate and disodium pamidronate. Recent studies have shown that these drugs delay progression of bony metastases and decrease the likelihood of bony fractures, and therefore women whose breast cancer has spread to the bone are often started on them.

Hormonal therapy

Hormonal therapy is used for women with HR-responsive tumours. The following drugs are used:

Anti oestrogens

Tamoxifen (Nolvadex®), toremifene, fulvestrant (Faslodex®)

Tamoxifen can be used for advanced breast cancer for women of any age if the cancer has recurred after the use of tamoxifen. If the cancer has recurred while on tamoxifen, a different drug is used. Toremifene is not often used because of its side effects. Fulvestrant is used for advanced breast cancer in post-menopausal women where the disease has progressed or there has been a relapse while on or after other anti-oestrogen therapy.

LHRH agonists

Goserelin (Zoladex®)

Goserelin is used to block the stimulus to the pituitary gland that in turn causes the ovaries to stop ovulating and producing oestrogen. It is used in pre-menopausal women. A potential side effect is osteoporosis, the risk of which may be minimized if given with tamoxifen.

Aromatase inhibitors

Anastrazole (Arimidex®), letrozole (Femara®), exemestane (Aromasin®)

These drugs block aromatase action and so reduce the production of oestrogen (see page 107). They are only suitable for post-menopausal women. Anastrazole and letrozole are effective treatments for metastatic breast cancer and are particularly beneficial for older women. They have fewer side effects than tamoxifen, including vaginal bleeding and blood clots, but there is a greater risk of osteoporosis and bone fractures. Exemestane is used for advanced breast cancer for women in whom other anti-oestrogen drugs have failed.

Progestogens

This group of drugs is only used as second- or third-line treatment now because there are different drugs that are more effective with fewer side effects.

Treatment for specific areas

Metastases in bone

The bone is the most common site for breast cancer metastases. Many patients with bone metastases have symptoms that are controlled well and they are able to have a good quality of life. A high calcium level in the blood (hypercalcaemia) is the most common derangement of metabolism from bony metastases and it can cause symptoms like nausea, abdominal pain, constipation, fatigue, confusion and drowsiness. The best treatment for this is rehydration (increased fluid intake) orally or intravenously (injected into a vein), and intravenous bisphosphonates (see page 130). This helps to flush the excess calcium out of the body.

Bony pain can also be managed with simple painkillers such as aspirin, or non-steroidal anti-inflammatory drugs, or opiate painkillers (for example, morphine). It is important to realize that pain can almost always be effectively managed so that patients are pain-free all of the time. Radiotherapy is the main treatment for localized bone pain. When there is more widespread, non-localized bone pain or recurrence of pain in an area previously treated with radiotherapy, bisphosphonates provide useful pain relief.

Isolated fractures or impending fractures of the long bones in the upper or lower limbs as a result of cancer deposits can sometimes be surgically fixed. Collapse of the vertebrae (spinal column bones) can cause spinal cord compression and urgent surgery or radiotherapy may be necessary to relieve compression of the spinal cord. Symptoms of spinal cord compression are pain around the spine, weakness, and a change in sensation in the legs. Rarely, breast cancer spreads to the bone marrow (bone marrow infiltration), where blood cells are produced. This can cause anaemia which leads to tiredness and breathlessness. Chemotherapy and hormonal therapy (for ER-positive tumours, see page 131) are used to treat bone marrow infiltration. Anaemia can be treated with blood transfusions.

Metastases in liver

Metastases in the liver can cause it to swell, and the stretching of the capsule around the liver can cause discomfort or pain. This is normally felt beneath the ribs or in the upper part of the abdomen. Sometimes the enlarged liver can cause pressure on the nerves that also go to the shoulder, and the shoulder may feel painful (referred pain). Hiccoughs can be caused by the pressure of the liver on the diaphragm, causing it to contract. The swelling associated with liver metastases can be reduced by corticosteroids (for example, dexamethasone). Painkillers are available for pain control. Nausea can be caused by the build-up of toxins normally processed by the liver or if there is pressure on the nearby stomach. Patients with liver metastases may lose their appetite. Eating small meals more frequently may be easier. Ascites (a collection of fluid in the abdomen) is sometimes a problem and the fluid may have to be drained to ease discomfort. This involves introducing a drainage tube into the abdominal cavity under local anaesthetic. Fluid is then allowed to drain off, usually over several hours before removal of the tube. If the fluid re-accumulates, the process can be repeated. Anaemia, jaundice and itching of the skin are also associated with liver metastases. Isolated liver metastases can sometimes be surgically removed but this is rare because, in most cases, several areas of the liver are affected. Other methods using ultrasound or lasers or the injection of substances that block the blood vessels to the tumours have been reported but are not often used.

Metastases in lung

Breathlessness is a common symptom of lung metastases. It can happen for a number of other reasons, including narrowing or blockage of the airways, a chest infection or feeling anxious. Narrowing of the airways may be treated with salbutamol (a drug that opens the airways) through an inhaler or nebulizer. A pleural effusion (a collection of fluid in the chest cavity) can also cause breathlessness. The fluid can be drained by introducing a drainage tube into the chest cavity. If the collection recurs and is troublesome, a sclerosing agent (for example, tetracycline, an antibiotic, bleomycin or talc) can be used that sticks the surfaces of the cavity together after drainage to obliterate the space. This procedure is called pleurodesis. A cough is a less common complaint that can be caused by irritation by the cancer itself or by an infection. Cough medicines or a saline (salt-water) nebulizer may help loosen any thick phlegm, making it easier to bring up. Pain is usually treated successfully with painkillers. Morphine may be necessary for pain or a cough. Loss of appetite, weight loss and tiredness are related to each other and can be caused by the cancer or the treatment. Eating small meals at frequent intervals may be tolerated better than normal meals.

Metastases in brain

Breast cancer very occasionally spreads to the brain. The most common symptom of brain metastases is a headache, which is often worse in the morning and gradually lessens during the day. Other symptoms include nausea, vomiting and fatigue, weakness (in general or down one side of the body), fits and double vision. Less commonly, there can be a change in behaviour, confusion and difficulty with speech. Radiotherapy is the most commonly used treatment for brain metastases. High-dose corticosteriod drugs can be used to relieve the symptoms of headache and nausea caused by pressure around the brain tumour. Isolated metastases can rarely be surgically removed, or treated with focused radiotherapy beams.

Clinical trials

The right treatment for breast cancer may not always be obvious, especially when women are faced with several options. There may be several tried and tested treatment methods, but new methods and drugs are emerging all the time. Sometimes the data is not available to provide all the answers and women may be asked if they would be willing to participate in a clinical trial.

A clinical trial is a proper scientific investigation that is carefully designed to answer a specific question. Standard treatment for breast cancer has evolved over many years of studying the different ways in which patients have responded to various treatments. Even so, a treatment that will cure all patients with breast cancer still does not exist. Therefore, new treatments are being sought all the time. When a new treatment method is found, doctors need to explore whether it will be more effective than standard treatment.

Participating in a trial has potential advantages:

- Patients may gain an added benefit with the new treatment compared to the standard treatment
- Patients will be given all the information they need to decide whether they agree to participate in the trial, and this may be more than they would receive otherwise
- Patients will probably receive more attention during treatment because the doctors and nurses will monitor the effects of the treatment and collect all the information
- It shows that the team is in contact with other breast cancer specialists and knows what treatment is being offered elsewhere and that they are working towards improving breast cancer treatment
- Most patients like being given the chance to make a contribution towards improving breast cancer treatment.

myth
Taking part in a clinical trial will mean that patients won't get properly treated.

fact
Patients can be reassured that if they take part in a clinical trial, they will not go without the treatment that their doctors feel they definitely should have. Some trials may involve a 'placebo' (dummy tablet or drug). If this is part of the trial it will mean that 'giving nothing' may be as good as the other treatment being investigated.

There are potential disadvantages:

- The new treatment may be found to be no better or even less effective than the standard treatment.
- It is often difficult for a patient to make a decision about whether or not to participate in a clinical trial.
- Extra visits to the hospital and extra tests may be necessary.

Patients who take part in a clinical trial make a very valuable contribution towards improving breast cancer treatment for patients of the future.

CHAPTER 5

Taking control

Living with a diagnosis of breast cancer will be a completely different experience for each woman. However, young or old, single or attached, with or without family or children, the initial diagnosis is a potentially devastating experience. Life does change. There is a whole host of decisions to be made. There are people to tell and arrangements to be made at home and at work. Sometimes, emotional support has to be given to others who are close. There is no one solution for how to best get through the situation. Getting through treatment can take several months, and it can take a year or two to get back into some sort of routine afterwards. A fear of the breast cancer returning and dreading the thought of maybe having to go through it all again are common.

my experience

In hospital wards and waiting rooms I met many women who were sharing my destiny, and I learned how very different our ways of coping with cancer were. Many wanted to share personal stories, but – while my treatment was going on – I felt that I didn't really want to hear them. Those whose treatment was successful seemed to me too upbeat about genuine risks. In other cases, where the cancer had progressed or returned, I was reminded of what I really didn't want to hear: there was a chance that the same thing would happen to me.

I soon developed strategies of avoiding such conversations but I also learned that there were many other women just like me, keen to discuss the latest play, a new restaurant or a handsome film star, keen not to give the cancer more precious time than was absolutely necessary, not to make it their destiny, whatever the final outcome. This did not mean that we were in denial, simply that we wanted to continue being mothers, lovers, teachers, writers, or whatever else we were before becoming cancer patients.

The impact on the partner and members of the family of a breast cancer patient is often underestimated. The partner of a breast cancer patient will often need to carry on in their job in order to provide financial support for the family, in addition to dealing with their own feelings about the breast cancer.

For those women living with advanced disease, the knowledge that breast cancer will be the probable cause of their death is something that others may not know how to react to and how to live with. Help is available from a variety of different sources. Breast care nurses attached to each breast unit can put women in touch with relevant organizations. There are contact details for some organizations on page 155.

Q I have just been told that I have breast cancer. How am I going to cope?

A Some women take things one step at a time. Others feel they would like to plan their whole course of treatment and decide on whether or not they will want surgery or chemotherapy or radiotherapy even before the results of the histology of the biopsy are known. It is probably best to liaise with your breast care nurse who will be able to explain each step of the process and give you advice and information along the way.

my experience

As a patient you have to get used to the fact that you will be talking to three different disciplines during your treatment – oncology, surgery and radiotherapy. I found that each one had a slightly different interpretation or slant on my situation. This can be confusing at first and for me it was important to keep a note of what was being said and to keep a list of questions that I needed to ask each person.

The different treatment choices that can be offered for local and systemic control of breast cancer are there for each women to question, consider and to choose or decline. The recommendation for treatment will usually be made by the multidisciplinary team of doctors and nurses that discusses each individual case. The team will give its recommendations according to information available at that time. The individual circumstance of each patient is carefully considered but the ultimate decision belongs to the patient. No one can force any treatment upon someone without his or her consent. A second opinion can be sought and is sometimes helpful to reinforce decision making. Seldom does a time delay in getting a second opinion affect an individual's outcome. Patients are encouraged to find out as much about their disease as they want by asking questions, and to participate in the management of their disease as much as they want.

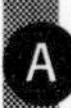

Q How do I tell my children that I have breast cancer?

A If you have more than one child, it is best to tell them all at the same time. Secrets tend to exclude. Be honest, brief and don't be afraid to use the word 'cancer'. Young children may become

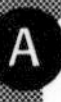

confused if you use euphemisms like 'lump'. They might think they need the treatment that you are going through if they bump their head and get a lump on their forehead. Explain your treatment plan and how it will be likely to affect you and your family.

Children of school age need support with their social life, school and out-of-school activities. Explain how much you will be able to participate in. Help them to recognize the difference between the side effects of your treatment and the effects of the disease. Talk about 'good days' and 'bad days', explain that you might need a good cry on a 'bad day'. Help them to recognize that illness isn't fair. Inform their teacher and the school nurse who will be able to put things into perspective at school.

Older children need help with balancing their time at home and with friends. Understand that relationships between teenagers and their parents are complex at the best of times. Daughters may be afraid of getting breast cancer themselves. Ask your breast care team about the risk to your family members.

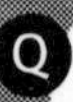

How will we cope as a family?

A Young children like their routine. If you need to make changes to their old routine, establish a new one as soon as you can. If you cannot participate in their care as much as before, try to make arrangements with someone else to whom they can look for consistency. Reassure them that they are not to blame for your illness.

Surgery

The section on surgery in Chapter 4 (page 64) explains surgical options for breast cancer excision and reconstruction. Here we look at hospital procedures and practical matters to help you deal with the day-to-day realities.

The hospital admission

On a practical level there are a number of things that are useful to bring to hospital:

- Toiletries
- Towel
- Pillow
- Pyjamas
- Dressing gown
- Bedroom slippers
- Portable music player
- Books and magazines
- Money (small change)
- Extra bra (non-wired)
- Change of clothes.

It is best not to bring valuable jewellery or a lot of money into hospital.

The admissions procedure is a little different at each hospital but women are normally sent a letter with instructions on where and when to go for registration. On the ward, details will be checked by a nurse and then a doctor, consent for the operation obtained and the operation site marked on the body.

For operations requiring a general anaesthetic, the patient is required to fast for several hours prior to the operation. It is helpful to know the approximate time at which the operation is scheduled in order to know when to stop eating and drinking. The anaesthetist (the doctor who gives the general anaesthetic or puts the patient to sleep) will usually pre-assess patients and explain the anaesthetic procedure to them before they are taken to the operating theatre department.

After the operation, it is normal for patients to spend some time in the recovery ward before being transferred back to their hospital ward. For complex operations, a period on a high-dependency unit may be necessary for more intensive monitoring before transfer back to the hospital ward. After a breast operation, it is usual for women to be up and about the day following their operation and to receive instruction by a physiotherapist on arm and shoulder movement, especially following surgery to the axilla (armpit). It is useful to have an instruction leaflet showing the exercises necessary to prevent stiffness of the shoulder. These are available from the breast care nurse or physiotherapist attached to the breast team.

Patients are normally allowed home when they have fully recovered from the anaesthetic and are mobile. Some women are allowed home with their drainage tubes in place but, more commonly, patients remain in hospital until the drains are removed. Patients should ask their doctors or nurses what the normal practice is in their unit. The amount of activity and movement that each patient will be expected to achieve or allowed to do will depend on the type of surgery performed. Women should ask their surgeon what is expected of them and whether they will be restricted from activities like driving a car, going back to work and doing housework or sporting activities. Sometimes the type of dressing applied to the wounds should not get wet. Some dressings are water-resistant and women may be allowed to shower or bathe with them on.

Before leaving hospital, it is useful for patients to obtain contact telephone numbers for their doctors or breast care nurse, and to ask who the best person is to get in touch with for any problems that might arise at home.

Patients are followed up in the outpatients' department usually between one to two weeks after discharge for a wound check, to get their histology results and to plan the next step of their treatment.

my experience

I found that there is another problem after the operation – when and how to show, or to conceal the damage done to your body so that your partner will not be scared, or get too stressed, or be 'put off' altogether. It is a highly individual problem, but I think it is helpful for women to learn how other breast cancer victims have dealt with the situation – after all, the range of possible actions and types of behaviour seems to be limited. My own solution was to wear a pretty, loose, silky camisole – not to expose the affected area to his gaze – and to wait for my partner to make his own decision about when he was willing and ready 'to take a look'. This worked well for me.

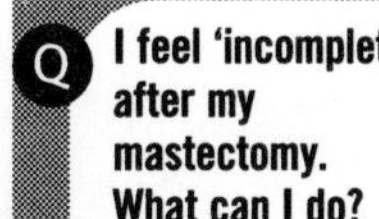

Q I feel 'incomplete' after my mastectomy. What can I do?

A Consider getting a breast reconstruction if you haven't had one. Ask your breast care nurse for an external breast prosthesis if you haven't already got one.

Q Can I travel after my treatment for breast cancer? How can I get travel insurance?

A Travel insurance may be obtained from your local travel agent, high street insurers or other insurance companies as listed by Breast Cancer Care (see page 155). It is worthwhile shopping around as the cost of premiums and the terms vary widely. Any claim relating to a pre-existing illness like breast cancer may not be covered if the insurance company is not informed when the policy is purchased. The cost of insurance varies according to which country you are travelling to (it is higher for the USA compared to Europe).

You may need a letter from your doctor confirming the details of your diagnosis and treatment, and declaring that you are fit to travel. For travel within the European Union (EU), reciprocal arrangements between countries exist if you need medical care while you are on holiday. You will need to fill in a form (E111) that is available from the post office, and have it stamped to take with you on holiday.

my experience

Following my mastectomy and reconstruction, my partner stayed with me throughout the recovery period and was there for me, sharing my pain, discomfort and distress, witnessing my wounds being dressed, drains being removed. I have not felt self-conscious and my partner has never found me less attractive.

my experience

Two areas of great importance and two 'guarantors' of coming back to life for me were the return to work and the return to an active sex life. I suppose it would be difficult, if not impossible, to get some useful advice about what, when and how to tell one's partner about 'the cancer experience', the fear and the gore, the pain and the sense of mutilation experienced in the aftermath of mastectomy. My personal decision was not to burden my partner with all the gory stories, and the pain suffered, but to give him some basic 'information' and see whether he wanted to know more, and whether he chose to ask more detailed questions. He did not, and that was fine by me.

Chemotherapy

A thorough discussion with the oncologist about the benefits and risks of chemotherapy and the types of drugs available for each individual patient is necessary. When the treatment is agreed, the procedure is explained and a consent form signed. Some patients may require a centrally placed catheter for the delivery of the drugs (for example, PICC, Portacath or Groshong line, see page 110). Combined chemotherapy regimes are commonly given in cycles lasting three to four weeks and six to eight cycles are given. Blood tests are taken before each cycle of chemotherapy in order to check the blood counts for anaemia or signs of lowered immune resistance, kidney function or liver function. Patients may be advised to take anti-nausea medications or steroids before the start of chemotherapy. The drugs are usually administered as an intravenous infusion (drip through a vein) lasting several minutes to several hours. They are usually given as a day case (the patient will not need to stay overnight in hospital). Specialist chemotherapy nurses administer the drugs.

myth

The more chemotherapy you have, the better the outcome.

fact

It is the combination of drugs at the right dose that will work best. Your oncologist will have carefully selected the drugs for your individual case, taking into account your particular type and stage of breast cancer, the function of your heart, liver, kidneys, your general health and any drugs that you have previously taken.

Q My treatment has caused vaginal dryness. What can I do?

A Vaginal moisturizers like Replens and Senselle provide moisture and help with irritation and discomfort. KY jelly, Sylk or Astroglide are soluble water-based products and act as lubricants during intercourse. They do not contain any hormones. Some women need a local oestrogen cream, tablet, pessary, or vaginal ring impregnated with oestrogen. These preparations should only be used at the lowest effective dose and the shortest effective time (not for more than three months at a time) because of the potential risk of the oestrogen promoting a growth effect on breast cancer. Discuss the risk of using these local oestrogen preparations with your oncologist.

my experience

Although you cannot take it all in at first, there is a wealth of support and back-up to help you get through the months of treatment. The personal support and encouragement that I received from the MacMillan adjuvant breast nurse at Charing Cross Hospital was invaluable. Having someone to phone about absolutely anything to do with my illness was very reassuring. I never felt concerned or worried about phoning Vanessa, whereas I would have been less inclined to contact the consultants outside of my appointments.

my experience

Now that the surgery is over and I have started with chemotherapy, I feel that I am extremely lucky in having the total support and help from my husband (in particular his nursing and physiotherapy skills), the practical and emotional help from my children and some very close friends. I have been deeply affected by the love and care shown, whether in practical help, phone calls, the 'get well' card or the simple written note which reminds me how much people care about me.

my experience

My husband will be going away for a few weeks in the middle of my course of chemotherapy. Rather than panicking, I have arranged for a dear friend who I haven't seen for a long time to stay with me. I know that we will laugh every day. I will get there in the end with her help.

Q Will I ever have a normal sex life again?

A Losing your hair and frequently being tired is not good for the libido. Having a painful scar, breast deformity or having lost a breast are other reasons for not being positive about your body image. The tiredness will pass. It will take some time to get over all the treatment. Your hair will grow back when chemotherapy is over. Scars normally grow red and lumpy, and then soften and become pale and less sensitive over time (some can take many months to settle down). Communicate with your partner. Let them know how you feel. Do this at a time that is unrelated to having sex. This eliminates the chance that you will feel tense and embarrassed. Try a different position during sex if your scar is sore. Try wearing comfortable or sexy nightwear if you are not comfortable with showing your body.

Q I have been treated for breast cancer and want to start a family. Will I put myself at risk if I become pregnant?

A For women who have been treated for breast cancer, pregnancy does not seem to be associated with a worse prognosis for their breast cancer. However the evidence to support this advice is relatively poor. Since most breast cancer recurrences appear within two or three years after the initial diagnosis, it is advisable to postpone pregnancy for about three years. You should have a full examination by your oncologist before attempting to become pregnant.

Radiotherapy

Following surgery, it is common to give chemotherapy and then radiotherapy if all three modalities are used. A consultation with the clinical oncologist is the first step. Occasionally radiotherapy is given instead of surgery as primary treatment. The course of radiotherapy treatment is explained and a consent form signed. A date for radiotherapy planning is given for a few weeks after surgery. It is helpful to have a good range of movements back in the shoulder and arm because the radiotherapy planning session involves the patient lying on the simulator machine for some time with their arm propped up on supports. This is so that images of the breast can be taken and the tumour bed and breast (or chest wall) can be targeted without the arm getting in the way. Tattoo marks are sometimes made on the skin of the chest wall to enable accurate positioning at each radiotherapy session.

When the treatment starts, it usually means attending the radiotherapy department every day on week days for about five or six weeks. The treatment lasts only a few minutes each time. The patient is carefully positioned on the treatment machine before treatment proceeds. Radiographers control the delivery of the radiotherapy remotely using controls outside the treatment room.

myth

Radiotherapy makes you feel sick and makes your hair fall out.

fact

Radiotherapy to the breast or chest wall does not cause nausea or hair loss. It is a local treatment and you may lose some of the hair at the lower part of the armpit or around the nipple. This myth about radiotherapy is confused with chemotherapy which can cause both nausea and hair loss.

myth

Radiotherapy makes you radioactive.

fact

External beam radiotherapy is most commonly used for breast cancer, and the treatment does not make you radioactive. If an implant is used, you will be admitted to hospital and treated in an isolated room for the duration of treatment. The radioactive implant will be removed before you are discharged, and you will not be radioactive.

When treatment is over

Patients receiving multimodality treatment of surgery, chemotherapy and radiotherapy can expect the treatment to last for many months. Some women have to make major adjustments to their lives. However, others do not find that that having breast cancer changes their lives

my experience

I found it was important to keep remembering that whatever life span Nature or the Almighty has allotted to us – nobody knows . . . Doctors can prolong our lives but they are not God to whom 'we owe our lives'. What they can do – and this is of tremendous importance – is to help us in our fight with illness and to assist us in our return to normal life, life which is worth living.

my experience

There are so many things that people say and that are in the news about cancer, which seem calculated to induce guilt. I decided to ignore them and follow only my doctors' advice. Other people may have other ideas. One of the most important things I've learned in the process is how to cope my way, to hear my own voice and know what I want.

much at all. Attending a follow-up consultation may suddenly bring back all the emotions that a woman experienced when she was first diagnosed or what she felt during treatment. It is normal to feel that way. While follow-up consultations are designed to monitor well-being and to look out for a recurrence of the breast cancer, most recurrences are found by women themselves in between the appointments. Women should therefore continue to be aware of their breast(s) and their bodies, and to report anything new that they are worried about. The breast care nurse on the team is usually a good person to contact for advice and will be able to co-ordinate appointments and any necessary investigations.

Coping with secondary cancer

Living with a diagnosis of metastatic breast cancer may be very difficult. Feelings of shock, fear, and sadness can be expected. The thought of going through treatment again may seem overwhelming. While some women prefer to cope with their emotions alone, others may benefit from support from MacMillan nurses, Marie Curie nurses, home care specialists or from hospice nurses. They are experienced in providing practical and emotional support at this difficult time. For long-term psychological support, a counsellor may be able to help. The organizations listed on page 155 can offer help and advice. Information about local support services is available from the breast care nurse on the team.

CHAPTER 6

Structure of the health care system

A diagnosis of breast cancer is usually made when a woman finds something in her breast that she is concerned about, or if an abnormality is seen on a screening mammogram. Women normally consult their General Practitioner (GP) in the first instance if they have a breast problem. If a breast cancer is suspected, GPs normally fax a referral to their local specialist breast unit so that the woman can be given an appointment within two weeks. Most district general hospitals and teaching hospitals run specialist breast clinics.

The National Health Service (NHS) Breast Screening Programme in the UK is recognized as one of the most effective and comprehensive in the world. Screening is recognized as an important method of detecting early breast cancers, the stage at which treatment is most likely to be curative. All women between the ages of 50–70 are invited for mammography every three years on the screening programme. Mammograms are carried out at a mobile unit or, less commonly, a fixed unit, and the films are read by radiologists in a breast screening centre.

Specialist breast clinic

Some private hospitals run Well Woman clinics that provide the services of a specialist breast clinic and include mammography. At the specialist breast clinic, there are many people with different roles:

Consultant (breast) surgeon

This is a doctor who specializes in breast surgery and usually has background training in general surgery. In the outpatient clinic, the consultant surgeon's role is to consult with the patient and to take a history, perform a clinical examination, order the necessary investigations and make a diagnosis. If a tissue diagnosis is necessary, he or she will do the FNA or core biopsy (see pages 53–4) or refer the patient to the radiologist if it needs to be done with image guidance. The surgeon will give the results of investigations and explain the recommended plan of management. The breast surgeon is commonly the breast team leader who facilitates and co-ordinates the running of the breast unit. He or she will perform surgery and provide follow-up care for patients.

Consultant oncoplastic breast surgeon

This is a doctor who specializes in breast surgery and reconstruction of the breast, commonly with background training in general surgery, less commonly with background training in plastic surgery. The role is the same as that of a consultant surgeon. In addition, they can perform reconstructive breast procedures, and some have training in aesthetic breast procedures.

Breast physician

This doctor specializes in the diagnosis and medical treatment of breast disease.

Clinical geneticist

A clinical geneticist specializes in inherited diseases. For breast cancer patients, a clinical geneticist will be able to calculate a woman's risk of breast cancer and arrange genetic testing if appropriate.

Associate specialist

This is a doctor who specializes in breast diagnostics or breast surgery, and who has not taken a formal training programme as set out by a Royal College and received a Certificate of Completion of Specialist Training (CCST). The role is similar to that of a consultant surgeon or breast physician but the consultant surgeon has overall responsibility for the associate specialist.

Clinical assistant

This is a doctor who has not taken a formal training programme in breast surgery. Their role is to assist the consultant surgeon or breast physician who is in overall charge. Most of the work of a clinical assistant is in the outpatient clinic.

Specialist registrar

This doctor is training on a programme set out by a Royal College with a view to obtaining a CCST. Their role is to cover many of the duties of a consultant who supervises their work.

Fellow in surgery

A fellow in surgery specializes in a particular branch of surgery at the end or close to the end of their training programme. In the UK, there are specific training fellowships in oncoplastic breast surgery aimed at surgeons in the last two years of their training programme. Their role is the same as a consultant surgeon who supervises their work.

Consultant radiologist

This is a doctor who specialises in imaging for diagnostic purposes. For example, a breast radiologist will read mammograms, perform image-guided (using ultrasound or mammography) biopsy or FNA, insert image-guided wires or coils for localization of tumours that cannot be felt, and perform ultrasound along with other imaging investigations.

Consultant histopathologist/cytologist

This doctor specializes in the examination of tissue/cells for diagnosis of disease. Such doctors are a core member of the multidisciplinary team and will have specialist experience relevant to breast pathology/cytology. His or her role is to provide a tissue/cell diagnosis so that treatment can be tailored to each individual patient. They study the specimens taken in the clinic (FNA or core biopsy) and tissue specimens that are removed at surgery.

Consultant oncologist

A consultant oncologist specializes in the treatment of cancer. Clinical oncologists provide expertise in radiotherapy and chemotherapy whereas medical oncologists give chemotherapy but do not practise radiotherapy. They prescribe treatment and provide follow-up care for patients.

Breast care nurse

Each breast unit usually has at least one nurse who is specially trained in the management of breast cancer and in the provision of information and advice. The nurses have counselling skills and provide emotional and psychological support, often acting as the patient's advocate. They provide information on lymphoedema and fit external breast form prostheses. They act to provide a co-ordinated and effective breast service. In some units nurse practitioners act as breast diagnosticians and run special nurse-led clinics.

Chemotherapy nurse specialist

This is a specially trained nurse who administers chemotherapy.

Diagnostic radiographer

A **diagnostic radiographer** is trained to take X-rays and has specific training and experience in mammography.

diagnostic radiographer
Person trained in the use of X-rays. (A therapeutic radiographer operates the equipment used to deliver radiotherapy for the treatment of cancer in a radiotherapy department.)

Ultrasonographer

This is a person who is trained and experienced in performing diagnostic ultrasound.

Clinic nurse

Clinic nurses co-ordinate the running of the breast clinic.

Health care assistant

This person assists in the running of the breast clinic.

Breast cancer common pathway

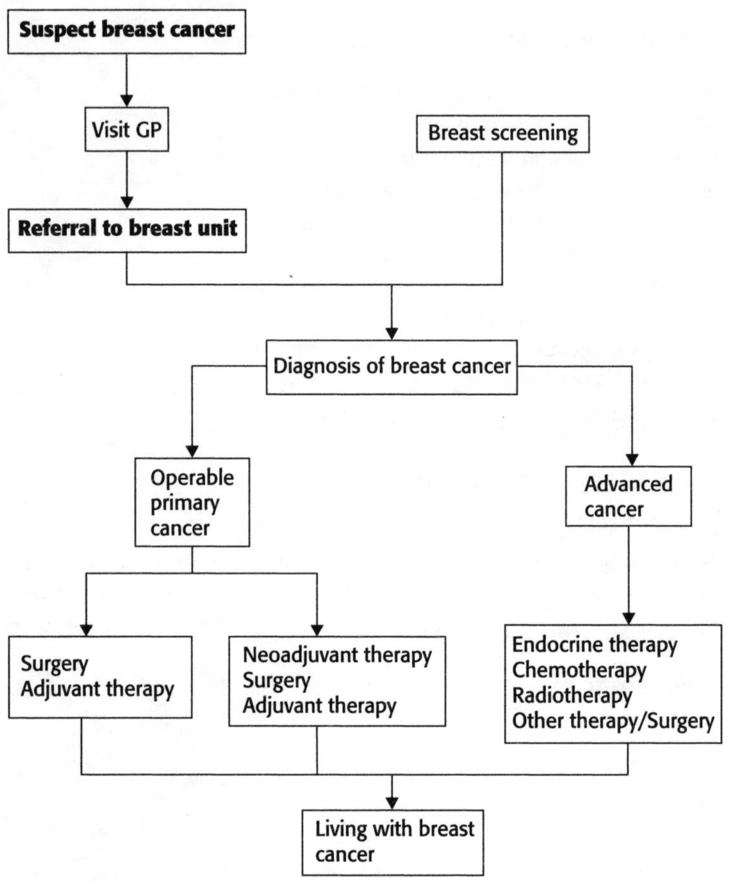

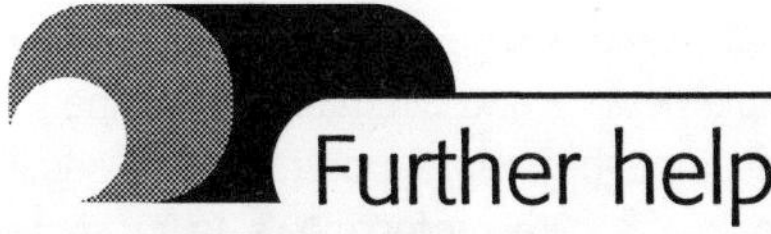

Further help

Breakthrough

Breakthrough is a charity and its aim is to raise awareness of breast cancer issues among the public and to campaign hard to keep breast cancer high on the media and political agendas. The charity has established a Research Centre for breast cancer research and treatment.

Weston House
3rd Floor
246 High Holborn
London WC1V 7EX
Telephone: 020 7025 2400
Fax: 020 7025 2401
Email: info@breakthrough.org.uk
www.breakthrough.org.uk

Breast Cancer Care

Breast Cancer Care is a charity and the UK's leading provider of information, practical assistance and emotional support for anyone affected by breast cancer, including younger women with breast cancer. Services are free.

Kiln House
210 New Kings Road
London SW6 4NZ (registered office)
Telephone: 020 7384 2984 (administration)
Fax: 020 7384 3387
Email: info@breastcancercare.org.uk
www.breastcancercare.org.uk

For a query of a medical nature, ring the free telephone helpline on 0808 800 6000, open Monday to Friday 09.00–17.00 and Saturday 09.00–14.00 or use the Ask the Nurse service. These services are only available to UK residents.

Breast Cancer Haven

Breast Cancer Haven is a charity that provides support centres for women with breast cancer. It provides complementary and alternative medicine to help heal the mind, body and spirit through group support and individual therapy programmes. It works with health care professionals to promote integrated breast cancer care.

Breast Cancer Haven
Telephone: 020 7384 0000

The London Haven
Telephone: 020 7384 0099

The Hereford Haven
Telephone: 01432 361 061
www.thehaventrust.org.uk

CancerBACUP

CancerBACUP was launched as a national cancer information service in October 1985. It provides high-quality and up-to-date information, practical advice and support with a free cancer information service staffed by qualified and experienced cancer nurses, publications on all aspects of cancer written specifically for patients and their families (available in full on the website), and a growing number of CancerBACUP local centres in hospitals up and down the country, also staffed by specialist cancer nurses.

CancerBACUP
3 Bath Place
Rivington Street
London EC2A 3JR

Telephone: 020 7696 9003
Switchboard open during office hours,
Monday–Friday, 09.00–17.30.
Fax: 020 7696 9002
www.cancerbacup.org.uk

Cancer information helpline (UK only)
Telephone: 0808 800 1234 (freephone)
Telephone: 020 7739 2280 (standard rate)
Lines staffed by cancer specialist nurses,
Monday–Friday, 09.00–20.00.
Please note: the old freephone number, 0800 181199, is no longer in use.

CancerHelp UK

CancerHelp UK is a free information service about cancer and cancer care for people with cancer and their families. It is brought to you by Cancer Research UK. It believes that information about cancer should be freely available to all and written in a way that people can easily understand.

Cancer Information Department
Cancer Research UK
P.O. Box 123
Lincoln's Inn Fields
London WC2A 3PX
Email (Cancerhelp UK secretary): sam.wiggins@cancer.org.uk
www.cancerhelp.org.uk

Cancer Research UK

The Cancer Research UK website has a wealth of information about the charity and about cancer.

P.O. Box 123
Lincoln's Inn Fields
London WC2A 3PX
Telephone (customer services): 020 7121 6699
Telephone (switchboard): 020 7242 0200
Fax: 020 7269 3100
www.cancerresearchuk.org

Macmillan

Macmillan Cancer Relief is a UK charity that works to improve the quality of life for people living with cancer. Macmillan offers life support by providing the expert care and practical support that makes a real difference to people living with cancer. They offer a range of innovative cancer services throughout the UK.

Macmillan CancerLine

Information or emotional support for patients and their family can be provided by contacting the Macmillan CancerLine:
Freephone: 0808 808 2020, 09.00–18.00 Monday–Friday.
Email: cancerline@macmillan.org.uk

Macmillan CancerLine
Macmillan Cancer Relief
89 Albert Embankment
London SE1 7UQ
www.macmillan.org.uk

A textphone service is available for the deaf and hard of hearing on 0808 808 0121.

Maggie's Centres

Maggie's Centres is a charitable organization for anybody who has, or who has had, cancer. It is also for their families, their friends and their carers. It provides centres close to a major cancer hospital treatment centre in order to allow people to take time out and to give them a non-institutional place they can call their own. The charity aims to help people with cancer to be as healthy in mind and body as possible and to enable them to make their own contribution to their medical treatment and recovery.

Maggie's Glasgow
The Gatehouse
Western Infirmary
10 Dumbarton Road
Glasgow G11 6PA
Telephone: 0141 330 3311
Fax: 0141 330 3363
Email: maggies.glasgow@ed.ac.uk
www.maggiescentres.org

Maggie's Edinburgh
The Stables
Western General Hospital
Crewe Road South

Edinburgh EH4 2XU
Telephone: 0131 537 3131
Fax: 0131 537 3130

Marie Curie Cancer Care

This is a charitable organization that provides care to thousands of cancer patients and their families, entirely free of charge. It provides community nursing care for terminally ill people, and has 10 hospices around the UK for care of patients and support of their carers. Referral to a hospice is usually arranged by a GP or hospital doctor. The Marie Curie Research Institute aids research in the investigation of the causes of cancer and better ways to treat the disease.

England

Marie Curie Cancer Care
89 Albert Embankment
London SE1 7TP
Telephone: 020 7599 7777
www.mariecurie.org.uk

Scotland

Marie Curie Cancer Care
29 Albany Street
Edinburgh EH1 3QN
Telephone: 0131 456 3700

Wales

Marie Curie Cancer Care
Raglan Chambers
63 Frogmore Street
Abergavenny
Monmouthshire NP7 5AN
Telephone: 01873 30 3000

Northern Ireland

Marie Curie Cancer Care
60 Knock Road
Belfast BT5 6LQ
Telephone: 028 9088 2060

National Cancer Institute

This is an American organization funded by the government that provides cancer-related health information and funding for scientific research throughout the USA. The Institute offers consumer-oriented information on a wide range of topics as well as descriptions of its research programmes for the general public and health professionals. Scientists will find detailed information on specific areas of research and funding opportunities. The Institute can be contacted directly for:

- Answers to questions about cancer
- Help with quitting smoking
- Informational materials
- Help using the website.

Telephone

To talk with an information specialist from the National Cancer Institute's Cancer Information Service – within the United States – Monday– Friday 09.00–16.30 local time:
1-800-4-CANCER
(1-800-422-6237)
TTY: 1-800-332-8615

Online (LiveHelp)

Use this feature for a confidential online text chat with an National Cancer Institute information specialist – Monday–Friday 9.00–11.00 US Eastern Time.

Email

For questions or comments on the website, use the online contact form.

Mail

Write to the National Cancer Institute at:
NCI Public Inquiries Office
6116 Executive Boulevard
Room 3036A
Bethesda, MD 20892-8322, USA
www.nci.nih.gov

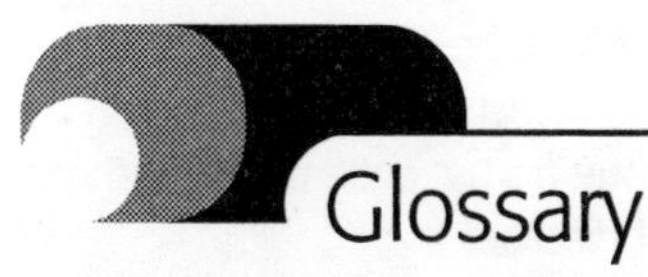

Glossary

Acini Tiny grape-shaped secretory portions of a gland.

Adenocarcinoma Cancer that arises in gland-forming tissue. Breast cancer is a type of adenocarcinoma.

Adjuvant systemic therapy Therapy such as chemotherapy or hormonal therapy that is given in addition to primary therapy (usually surgery).

Advanced breast cancer The cancer has metastasized (spread) to other parts of the body through the bloodstream or has become very large and spread into the skin or muscles of the chest wall (locally advanced).

Amenorrhoea Absence or stoppage of menstrual period.

Anorexia Loss of appetite.

Anthracyclines A group of cytotoxic antibiotic drugs that include doxorubicin and epirubicin among others. Mitoxantrone (mitozantrone) is a derivative of this group.

Anti-inflammatory drug Drug that reduces inflammation. Common examples are paracetamol or ibuprofen (Nurofen®).

Areola Pigmented skin around the nipple.

Aspiration Use of a hypodermic needle into a tissue to draw out fluid or cells.

Asymmetry Imbalance.

Atypical ductal hyperplasia Cells lining a breast duct that are slightly abnormal and increased in number.

Atypical lobular hyperplasia Abnormal cells within a breast lobe that are increased in number but fill less than half of the acini.

Autologous From the same person.

Axilla Armpit.

Axillary dissection Removal of lymph glands from the armpit.

Axillary nodes Lymph glands in the armpit.

Axillary sampling Removal of a few lymph glands from the armpit.

Benign Non-cancerous.

Bilateral Involving both sides.

Bilateral prophylactic mastectomy Surgical removal of both breasts in order to reduce the risk of a breast cancer.

Biopsy Examination of tissue from a patient for diagnosis, extent or cause of disease.

Bone marrow Soft inner part of bones that produces blood cells.

Bone scan Examination that looks for signs of cancer spread to bone.

BRCA1 gene Breast cancer susceptibility gene that has been linked to breast cancer in certain families. There is also an increased risk of ovarian, bowel and prostate cancer.

BRCA2 gene Breast cancer susceptibility gene that has been linked to breast cancer in certain families. There is also an increased risk of ovarian, prostate and pancreatic cancer.

Breast conserving surgery Surgery to remove the tumour with a rim of normal surrounding tissue as opposed to mastectomy (removal of the whole breast).

Breast reconstruction Surgical procedure to rebuild a natural looking breast shape after mastectomy.

Calcification Small calcium deposits in the body that can be seen on an X-ray.

Capsular contracture Formation of a very thick fibrous capsule that can cause pain and deformity of the breast in extreme cases.

Capsule Fibrous tissue that forms around any foreign material that is inserted into the body.

Carcinoma	Cancer arising from epithelial tissue (skin, glands, lining of internal organs). Breast cancer commonly arises from the lining of the breast lobular-ductal unit.
Cellulitis	Soft tissue infection.
Chemotherapy	Treatment of cancer using anti-cancer drugs to destroy cancer cells.
Clear margin	When a cancer is excised, it is sent to be examined under the microscope to ensure that the whole tumour has been removed with a rim of healthy tissue around it. This is to ensure that no tumour is left behind.
Clinical trial	Carefully planned and controlled study using volunteers to test new treatments, techniques or medical products.
Connective tissue	Supporting or framework tissue of the body (for example fat, elastic tissue, cartilage, bone).
Contracture	Formation of thick scar tissue, for example, around a breast implant.
Contralateral tumour	Tumour in the opposite breast to the one with breast cancer.
Core (needle) biopsy	A type of thick needle biopsy where a small core of tissue is removed from an area in the breast without surgery.
CT (Computerized axial Tomography) scan	A radiological test where multiple X-rays are taken and where a computer processes the images to give a detailed picture of the presence, size and position of a tumour.
Cyst	Fluid-filled sac.
Cystosarcoma phylloides	Breast tumour with variable malignant potential.
Cytological examination	Examination (by a specialist doctor) of cells under the microscope in order to make a diagnosis.
Cytologist	Specialist doctor who studies cells.
Cytology	Branch of medicine concerned with the study of the structure and function of cells.
Cytotoxic drug	Drug that kills an actively dividing cell.
Diagnostic radiographer	Person trained in the use of X-rays. A therapeutic radiographer operates the equipment used to

	deliver radiotherapy for the treatment of cancer in a radiotherapy department.
DIEP flap	Deep Inferior Epigastric artery Perforator flap – flap from the patient's own lower abdominal tissue that does not contain any muscle.
DNA	Deoxyribonucleic acid. Genetic code.
Donor site	Area from where tissue (for example skin, fat or a flap) is taken.
Drain	A surgical tube inserted at operation to remove fluids that accumulate in the operated area after the operation.
Duct	Vessel for conveying glandular secretions or lymph.
Ductal carcinoma in situ (DCIS)	Non-invasive cancer arising from breast ducts.
Dysplasia (of cells)	Abnormality in development giving rise to abnormal cell size, shape and organization.
Endocrine therapy	Drugs used to counter the effects of natural hormones on cancer.
Endogenous oestrogen	Oestrogen that is produced within the woman's own body.
Exogenous oestrogen	Oestrogen from an external source like the contraceptive prill or HRT.
Expander	Inflatable implant.
Flap	A portion of tissue that is moved (while still maintaining its blood supply) from one part of the body to another.
Free flap	A flap that is removed from one part of the body and transferred to another part of the body where its blood vessels are microsurgically connected to nearby vessels in order to receive a blood supply.
Gammalinoleic acid (GLA)	The active ingredient in evening primrose oil or starflower oil that helps in the management of breast pain.
Gene	Sequence of DNA required to produce a protein.
Gynaecomastia	Male breast enlargement.
Haematoma	Collection of blood beneath the skin.
Haemorrhage	Bleeding.
Herceptin	A drug also known as 'trastuzumab'. It is an antibody that sticks on to a certain protein called

	HER2, found in some cancers, and causes them to stop growing.
Histopathologist	An expert in the branch of medicine relating to clinical diagnosis of disease using laboratory methods.
Hodgkin's disease	A type of cancer involving the lymph nodes.
Hormone	Chemical substance produced by glands that enters the bloodstream and affects other organs.
Hormone Replacement Therapy (HRT)	Drugs containing oestrogen with or without progesterone that are used to treat symptoms of menopause.
Hyperplasia	Increase in the number of normal cells in a tissue.
Immune system	The body's system for fighting against a foreign attack.
Incision biopsy	Operation involving removal of part of a lump or tissue for diagnosis.
Infiltrating cancer	Cancer that invades into neighbouring tissue. It does not imply systemic spread.
In situ	Within the original confines. An in-situ cancer does not invade beyond the site of origin or into neighbouring tissue.
Internal mammary nodes	Lymph glands behind the edge of the sternum (breastbone).
Intraductal	Within the duct.
Intravenously	Injection into a vein.
Invasive cancer	Infiltrating cancer.
Latissimus dorsi (LD) flap	Large muscle (with or without skin) flap that can be used for reconstruction after mastectomy or partial mastectomy.
Latissimus dorsi (LD) muscle	Large muscle covering the surface of the back.
LHRH agonist	A drug that mimics Luteinizing Hormone Releasing Hormone (LHRH) thereby reducing the amount of circulating oestrogen in the body.
Lobular carcinoma in situ (LCIS)	Abnormal cells within the breast lobule (part of the breast capable of producing milk) that fill, distend, and distort more than half the acini of a breast lobule. This serves as a marker for future breast cancer risk.

Lobule	Part of the breast that is capable of producing milk.
Loco-regional recurrence	Recurrence of breast cancer in the breast or lymph nodes in the axilla, supraclavicular fossa (area above the collar bone) or internal mammary nodes (behind and beside the breast bone).
Lumpectomy	Surgical removal of a lump with a rim of normal tissue around it.
Lymph	Tissue fluid.
Lymph node	Lymph gland.
Lymphatic vessel	Vessels that carry lymph to and from lymph nodes.
Lymphoedema	Swelling of the arm, breast or chest wall that is caused by an accumulation of lymph in the tissues.
Lymphovascular invasion	Cancer cells have invaded tiny lymph channels or blood vessels in the tissue surrounding the tumour.
Malignant	A tumour that is able to spread and grow in other parts of the body (metastasize).
Mammography	X-ray examination of the breasts.
Mastectomy	Surgical removal of the breast.
Mastitis	Infection or inflammation of the breast.
Mastopexy	Surgical uplift of the breast.
Menarche	Age at which menstruation or a woman's periods starts.
Menopause	'Change of life', the time in a woman's life when her periods stop and her ovaries stop producing oestrogen.
Metastases	Appearance of cancer in parts of the body outside the original organ. Breast cancer can metastasize to the lungs, liver, bone or brain but rarely to other places.
Metastasis	Spread of cancer to a different organ, usually through the bloodstream to form secondary cancers (metastases).
Microcalcification	Tiny calcium deposits in the body that can be seen on an X-ray. Microcalcifications seen on a mammogram can sometimes signify DCIS.
Micrometastases	Small groups of cells that have left the original organ that are not clinically detectable.

Micrometastasis	Microscopic spread of cancer cells to other organs.
MRI scan or NMR scan	Magnetic Resonance Imaging or Nuclear Magnetic Resonance scan used to image soft tissues including the breast.
Multidisciplinary care	Combination of care from different specialists.
Multifocal disease	More than one diseased area.
Multifocal tumour	More than one tumour.
Multimodality treatment	The use of different forms of treatment. For breast cancer, surgery, drug therapy and radiotherapy are used.
Neoadjuvant therapy	Additional therapy that is given before surgery.
Nipple–areola complex	The nipple with its surrounding dark pigmented skin.
Oncogene	Tumour gene present in the body that can be activated and cause cells to grow and divide in an uncontrolled manner.
Oncologist	Specialist doctor in the treatment of cancer.
Oncoplastic technique	Surgical technique combining both surgical specialities of cancer surgery for excision of the tumour (onco) and plastic surgery (plastic) for reconstruction.
Osteoporosis	Softening of the bones and bone loss that occurs with increasing age in some people.
Ovarian ablation or suppression	Suppression of oestrogen production by the ovaries or surgical removal of the ovaries.
Palliation	Act of relieving a symptom without affecting the cause.
Pathologist	An expert in the branch of medicine relating to clinical diagnosis of disease using laboratory methods.
Pectoralis muscle	Muscle that lies on the front of the chest wall. Pectoralis major is the large muscle and pectoralis minor the small one.
Pedicled flap	Flap of tissue (skin, muscle or fat or a combination) that is attached to its original blood supply.
Port (of expander implant)	Reservoir that is attached to the expander. It allows the injection of saline (salty water) into the expander.

Post-menopausal After the menopause.

Progesterone Hormone produced in the ovary involved in the menstrual cycle and during pregnancy.

Prognosis Forecast of the expected or probable outcome of a disease.

Prosthesis Artificial substitute for a missing body part.

Protocol Detailed plan of a procedure, test or trial.

Quadrantectomy Surgical removal of a quarter of the breast.

Radial scar A radial scar is a benign (non-cancerous) area of fibrous tissue surrounded by breast glands, some of which may look abnormal under the microscope. On a mammogram a radial scar has the appearance of having long spicules (strands) radiating from a central area. A lump is not usually palpable in the breast.

Radiation therapy Radiotherapy using high energy rays like X-rays or photons.

Radiographer (for mammography) Person who operates the X-ray equipment and takes X-rays of the breast.

Recurrence Regrowth.

Sarcoma Cancer arising in the connective tissue.

Segmentectomy Surgical removal of a segment of the breast.

Sentinel node biopsy Surgical removal of the sentinel node.

Sentinel node of the breast The first node receiving lymphatic drainage from the breast. It is frequently in the lower part of the axilla.

Seroma Collection of tissue fluid beneath the skin.

Side effect Undesirable effect as a result of treatment that is not intentional.

Silicone Synthetic material used in the medical industry as a lubricant or in breast implants as a gel filler or shell.

Stereotactic guidance When an area of concern is seen on a mammogram and it is non-palpable (cannot be felt) and cannot be seen on an ultrasound scan, it can be sampled using X-ray control. This method is called stereotactic guidance and it can be used to pinpoint the exact location of a lesion by using information from mammograms taken

	from two different angles that is fed into a computer.
Supraclavicular	Area above the collar bone.
Systemic	Affecting the whole body.
Systemic therapy	Therapy affecting the whole body.
Tamoxifen	Drug that blocks oestrogen receptors on the cell surface.
Tietze's syndrome	Inflammation of the costal cartilage (at the junction between the rib(s) and the breast bone).
TP53	A cancer gene also known as tumour protein p53 (Li-Fraumeni syndrome). It is a tumour suppressor gene and acts by regulating the cycle of cell division by preventing cells from dividing and growing in an uncontrolled way.
TRAM flap	Transverse Rectus Abdominis Muscle flap – flap from the patient's own lower abdominal tissue that includes muscle.
Wide local excision or lumpectomy	Surgical removal of the lump with a wide (usually about 1 cm) margin of normal tissue surrounding the tumour.

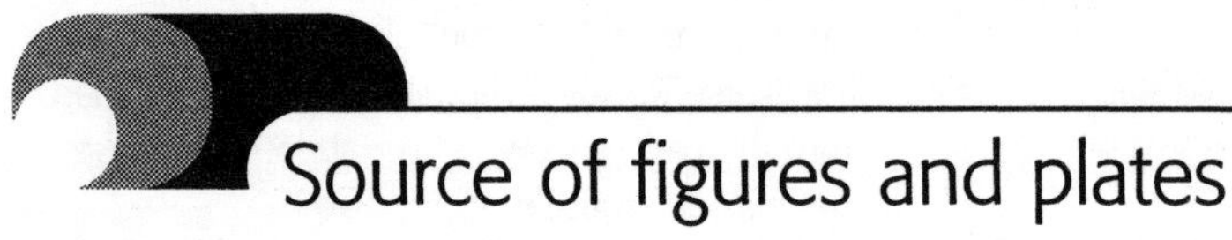

Source of figures and plates

Figure 1
Anatomy of the normal breast.

Figure 2
Microscopic anatomy of normal duct, ductal carcinoma in situ (DCIS) and invasive cancer.

Figure 3
Survival curve according to stage of breast cancer. (Cancer Research UK: Breast Cancer Factsheet – February 2004).

Figure 4
Types of lump versus age. (*Guideline for referral of patients with breast problems*, second edition, NHS Breast Screening Programme.)

Figure 5
Surgery for primary breast cancer.

Figure 6
Levels of axillary clearance.

Figure 7
Sentinel node biopsy.

Figure 8
Breast reconstruction using an implant expander.

Figure 9
Breast reconstruction with latissimus dorsi flap.

Figure 10
Breast reconstruction with abdominal flap.

Colour Plate 1
Normal breast tissue – appearance under the microscope. Cross section of a duct lined by normal ductal cells. (Courtesy of Professor Sami Shousha.)

Colour Plate 2
Ductal carcinoma in situ (DCIS is shown in red and the normal ducts are shown in yellow). Computer-Assisted Three-Dimensional Reconstruction of the Mammary Ductal/Lobular Systems. CANCER, Vol. 91, No. 12, 2001, pp. 2263–72. Copyright © 2001 American Cancer Society. Reprinted by permission of Wiley-Liss Inc., a subsidiary of John Wiley & Sons Inc.

Colour Plate 3
Ductal carcinoma in situ – appearance under the microscope. Cross section of a duct filled with abnormal ductal cells. (Courtesy of Professor Sami Shousha.)

Colour Plate 4
Left breast cancer showing breast asymmetry.

Colour Plate 5
Left breast cancer showing skin puckering beneath left breast when arms are raised. (Same patient as in Colour Plate 4.)

Colour Plate 6
Immediate partial breast reconstruction with latissimus dorsi flap after left hemi-mastectomy (volume replacement oncoplastic technique). (Same patient as in Colour Plates 4 and 5.)

Colour Plate 7
Inversion/retraction of right nipple (associated in this case with right breast cancer).

Colour Plate 8
Blood stained nipple discharge (associated in this case with ductal carcinoma in-situ and microinvasion).

Colour Plate 9
Mammographic appearance of a spiculate mass. In this case showing left breast cancer.

Colour Plate 10

Ultrasound appearance of an irregular solid mass. In this case showing left breast cancer.

Colour Plate 11a

Breast conserving surgery (central wide local excision) and radiotherapy for right breast cancer.

Colour Plate 11b

After right nipple–areola reconstruction with nipple share and tattoo technique.

Colour Plate 12

Immediate breast reconstruction with latissimus dorsi flap following right skin-sparing mastectomy.

(a) Preoperative appearance – the dotted lines show mid-line and extent of breast tissue to be excised, continuous lines are incision lines.
(b) Skin marks showing plan for latissimus dorsi flap.
(c) Three weeks after surgery – nipple-areola skin replaced by skin from back.
(d) Three weeks after surgery – latissimus dorsi donor scar on the back.

Colour Plate 13

Immediate breast reconstruction with implant expander and prosthetic nipple–areola complex following right mastectomy.

Colour Plate 14

Immediate partial breast reconstruction with latissimus dorsi flap after right upper hemi-mastectomy (volume replacement oncoplastic technique).

Colour 15

Immediate breast reconstruction with free abdominal deep inferior epigastric artery perforator (DIEP) flap after left mastectomy.

Colour Plate 16

A patient receiving external beam radiotherapy after breast conserving surgery for breast cancer.

Colour Plate 17

A patient receiving chemotherapy following surgery for breast cancer.

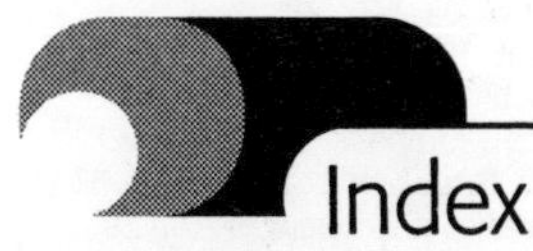

Index

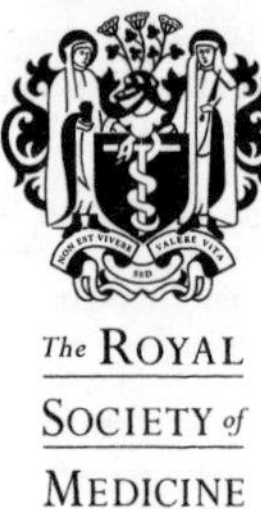

The Royal Society of Medicine (RSM) is an independent medical charity with a primary aim to provide continuing professional development for qualified medical and health-related professionals. The public benefits from health care professionals who have received high quality and relevant education from the RSM.

The Society celebrated its bicentenary in 2005. Each year it arranges and holds over 400 meetings for health care professionals across a wide range of medical subjects. In order to aid education and training further the Society also has the largest postgraduate medical library in Europe – based in central London together with online access to specialist databases. RSM Press, the Society's publishing arm, publishes books and journals principally aimed at the medical profession.

A number of conferences and events are held each year for the public as well as members of the Society. These include the successful 'Medicine and me' series, designed to bring together patients, their carers and the medical profession. In addition the RSM's Open and History of Medicine Sections arrange meetings on a regular basis which can be attended by the public.

In addition to the lectures and training provided by the RSM, members of the Society also have access to club facilities including accommodation and a restaurant. The conference and meeting facilities of the RSM were refurbished for their bicentenary and are available to the public for hire for meetings and seminars. In addition, Chandos House, a beautifully restored Georgian townhouse, designed by Robert Adam, is also now available to hire for training, receptions and weddings (as it has a civil wedding licence).

To find out more about the Royal Society of Medicine and the work it undertakes please visit www.rsm.ac.uk or call 020 7290 2991. For more information about RSM Press, please visit www.rsmpress.co.uk.